The Supervisor Training Curriculum

The Supervisor Training Curriculum

Evidence-Based Ways to Promote Work Quality and Enjoyment Among Support Staff

Dennis H. Reid
Marsha B. Parsons
Carolyn W. Green

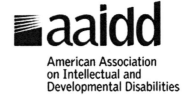

American Association on Intellectual and Developmental Disabilities

Acknowledgment

We express our sincere appreciation to the many dedicated supervisors with whom we have worked who continuously strive to help their staff provide high-quality services for people with intellectual disabilities. We also acknowledge those applied researchers who have validated effective means of training and supervising the performance of support staff in human service agencies. Without the accomplishments of these dedicated professionals, the development of an evidence-based curriculum for training supervisors would not have been possible.

Copyright © 2011 by Habilitative Management Consultants, Inc.

Published by
American Association on Intellectual and Developmental Disabilities
501 3rd Street, NW Suite 200
Washington, DC 20001-2760

Printed in the United States of America

Library of Congress Cataloging-in-Publication Data

Reid, Dennis H.
 The supervisor training curriculum : evidence-based ways to promote work quality and enjoyment among support staff / Dennis H. Reid, Marsha B. Parsons, Carolyn W. Green.
     p. cm.
  ISBN 978-1-935304-08-1 (alk. paper)
 1. Human services personnel—Supervision of—United States. 2. Social work with people with disabilities—United States. 3. People with disabilities—Services for—United States. 4. Human services personnel—Training of. 5. Supervisors—Training of—United States. I. Parsons, Marsha B. II. Green, Carolyn W. III. American Association on Intellectual and Developmental Disabilities. IV. Title.
  HV40.54.R455 2011
  362.3068'4—dc22
                              2010051729

Preface

The Supervisor Training Curriculum is a curriculum for training supervisors, and prospective supervisors, in evidence-based means of training, supervising, and motivating support staff. The curriculum is designed for supervisors working in, or going to work in, any setting providing supports and services for people with intellectual and related disabilities. The content is based on the results of over three decades of applied research on staff training and supervision and the authors' corresponding amount of supervisory experience. The curriculum methodology is performance based and competency based, requiring trainees to successfully master both classroom and on-the-job performance criteria to complete the training.

Contents

Part I: Introduction 1

    Using *The Supervisor Training Curriculum* 3

    Introducing the Training Process 6

Part II: Training Modules 7

    Module 1: Introduction to Supervision 9

    Module 2: Making Performance Expectations Clear:
                  Specifying Work Duties 15

    Module 3: Making Performance Expectations Clear:
                  Job Duty Checklists 23

    Module 4: Assessing Work Performance: Formal Monitoring 33

    Module 5: Assessing Work Performance: Informal Monitoring 47

    Module 6: Improving and Supporting Work Performance:
                  Diagnostic Feedback 57

    Module 7: Staff Training 69

    Module 8: Promoting Quality Work Performance With Enjoyment 83

    Module 9: Reducing Workplace Discontent 97

    Module 10: Resolving Recurrent Performance Problems 109

    Module 11: Putting It All Together:
                   Improving Selected Areas of Staff Performance 123

Part III: On-the-Job Competency Checks:
           Trainer Instructions and Forms 135

Part IV: Selected Background Readings 141

Part I

Introduction

Using *The Supervisor Training Curriculum*

The Supervisor Training Curriculum consists of two primary parts. The first part is the curriculum proper, to be used by trainers when training supervisors. The second part is the *Trainee Guide*. The guide is to be given to trainees as a resource and a note-taking tool.

The curriculum consists of 11 training modules. Each module is organized into 5 basic parts:

1. Module introductory sheet
2. Presentation summary
3. Visual aids
4. Activity sheets
5. Competency checks

Each of these parts is summarized in subsequent sections.

The curriculum is designed to be carried out by two trainers with a respective group of trainees. Generally, it is best that each training group have at least 2 trainers and no more than 25 trainees. With smaller groups of trainees, one trainer can conduct the training with the curriculum. However, that trainer would need to solicit the assistance of one or more trainees to help with role-play demonstrations that are usually conducted by two trainers.

The amount of time typically needed to train each module within the curriculum is designated in the respective module introductory sheet. In total, the training encompasses two days of classroom training for each group of trainees. The training can be grouped within two days, with Modules 1 through 6 being trained on the first day and Modules 7 through 11 being trained on the second day. Alternatively, the training could be broken down into shorter classroom training periods to accommodate trainer and trainee schedules (e.g., in 2-hour training blocks, with one block per day). Additionally, approximately 45 minutes is required with each trainee in the trainee's routine work setting in order for the trainer to conduct competency checks as part of the on-the-job training. It is recommended that, when possible, the on-the-job training component be conducted after classroom training with Module 6 has been completed and before classroom training is resumed with Module 7. However, the on-the-job training can also be conducted after all the classroom training is completed.

Module Introductory Sheet

Each module introductory sheet identifies the skills to be taught in the module, the objectives to be mastered by trainees, the general procedures and processes to be used in the training, the types of competency checks to be used to assess trainee mastery, the estimated amount of time to train with the module, and the necessary materials for training.

Presentation Summary

The presentation summary represents the core content of each module. It presents the procedures, processes, and content of each module in a step-wise fashion. The summary delineates the topics the trainers should present and describe, the demonstrations to be provided, and the activities to be completed by trainees. The summary is organized to facilitate the training process by providing highlighted pointers to trainers next to the detailed instructions in the summary proper. These pointers are provided in the left margin next to the corresponding text information.

More detailed instructions to trainers (e.g., how to conduct activities, when to ask specific questions) are separated from the text to be presented by trainers by a different font and horizontal lines as indicated in the following illustration.

Instructions to trainers are presented in the following format:

When you see this font between two lines, the information is for the trainer's use only (i.e., the information is not to be presented to trainees).

For effective training with the curriculum, it is essential that trainers become extremely familiar with all parts of the presentation summary. It is also essential that trainers practice the demonstrations and learning activities within each module prior to conducting training sessions and have available all necessary materials as indicated on the module introductory sheet (e.g., copies of activity sheets and competency check forms).

Within the modules, a heavy emphasis is placed on trainer demonstration of target skills and trainee practice of the skills. As trainees practice various skills with the activities described in the presentation summary, trainers must continuously circulate among the trainees to observe their practice activities, answer trainee questions, and provide supportive and corrective feedback as needed. No trainee activity or competency check should be considered completed until trainers have observed each trainee complete the activity or check proficiently. Guidelines for evaluating trainee proficiency are provided at the end of the chapters containing competency checks as well as in the Competency Check section (part III) of the curriculum.

Visual Aids

Visual aids are used during training. A website (see inside front cover) is provided that offers a PowerPoint presentation for trainer use with each module. The slides are arranged in the order in which they are to be used within each module. Additionally, immediately following each module's presentation summary are paper copies of the slides. These may be reproduced as overhead transparencies. Depending on whether the slides or overhead transparencies are used, a computer and digital projector or overhead transparency projector will be needed, respectively.

Activity Sheets for Trainee Use

Activity sheets are used during training. Most modules contain activity sheets for trainee practice of various skills. The activity sheets are arranged in the order in which they are used with each module (located immediately after the paper copies of the slides for each module).

Competency Checks

Competency checks are used to ensure trainees demonstrate skill mastery of the training content. Each trainee must successfully complete module competency checks to be certified as having completed the training. The competency checks are designed to assess a variety of knowledge and skills related to evidence-based supervision. There are four types of competency checks: (a) quiz questions, (b) in-class activities, (c) in-class role-play demonstrations, and (d) on-the-job demonstrations.

The competency checks are described at the end of each module, along with trainer instructions for administering the checks. The mastery criteria for completing each competency check are included with the instructions for the trainers. Competency check forms are also included at the end of each module for checking trainees' competency. A separate packet of trainer instructions and forms for the on-the-job competency checks is provided in part III of the curriculum. The latter competency checks are intended to be conducted within one day for each trainee at the trainee's regular job site.

To facilitate using the competency checks to assess trainee mastery of the curriculum content, it is helpful if trainers divide up the trainees in each class. Each trainer should be responsible for checking the competency of all trainees in his or her respective group.

Introducing the Training Process

The presentation summary for each module provides specific information for presenting each module. Most of the modules emphasize teaching performance skills related to evidence-based supervision. As such, many modules involve trainer demonstrations and trainee practice activities conducted in role-play situations. Because some trainees are likely to feel awkward when initially required to demonstrate various skills during the role plays, it is important for trainers to address this issue early in the training process. Trainers should inform trainees they will practice performing a number of skills and that feeling awkward at first is to be expected and is certainly acceptable. Trainees should be further informed that the initial awkwardness that they might experience typically goes away after a few activities.

To facilitate the trainees to be comfortable with the role-play activities, trainers should make special attempts to praise the efforts of trainees during the role plays. The training process is also designed to minimize initial difficulty with trainee role-play demonstrations by having the trainers first display the skills of concern themselves.

It is critical to explain the purpose of the demonstrations and role-play activities. It should be emphasized that to truly learn to perform the skills involved in evidence-based supervision, trainees must have opportunities to practice and receive feedback on the application of the skills in as lifelike a situation as possible. Hence, a number of role-play activities will be conducted in which trainers and trainees role-play a supervisor, a support staff person, and a client with a disability. It *must* be explained that by role-playing the part of a staff member or a client with a disability, the intent is by no means to be condescending toward support staff or people with disabilities. Rather, the intent is to make the practice situation as similar to the trainee's work situation as possible. To make the situation as lifelike as possible, trainees must practice the skills in situations they are likely to encounter with support staff and agency clients. That is the only reason trainers and trainees will be role-playing the part of a support staff person or client.

Part II

Training Modules

MODULE 1

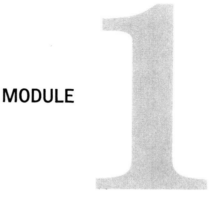

Introduction to Supervision

The following will be covered on day 1 of training.

Objectives

Upon completion of this module, trainees should be able to do the following:

1. Identify the two main components of a supervisor's job.
2. Identify the three goals of this training for supervisors.
3. Describe an evidence-based approach to supervision and its accompanying benefits.

Method

1. Presentation on introduction to the training: *2 minutes*
2. Trainee question-and-answer activity: *8 minutes*
3. Presentation and trainee discussion on the job of a supervisor: *10 minutes*
4. Presentation and trainee discussion on the goals of this training for supervisors: *10 minutes*
5. Presentation on evidence-based supervision: *5 minutes*

Competency Check, Materials, and Total Training Time

1. Competency check: Mastery completion of comprehensive modules' quiz (administered after Module 7)
2. Materials
   a. PowerPoint presentation equipment (LCD, computer, curriculum CD) or
   b. Overhead projector and copies of Slides 1.1, 1.2, 1.3, and 1.4
3. Total training time: *35 minutes*

Introduction to Supervision

INTRODUCE SUPERVISION

This is the first in a series of classes on supervision. In this and the classes to follow, we will be talking about, demonstrating, and practicing effective ways to supervise the work performance of support staff. We will focus on how to assist the staff in providing the best supports and services possible for people with disabilities.

Supervising the work performance of support staff is a process that is often misunderstood. Although there are several reasons why confusion exists about how to supervise, there is one very common reason. Let us do an activity that illustrates this reason.

QUESTION TRAINEES

Ask trainees to think about when they were children and about what they wanted to be when they grew up. Then ask three or four trainees to share with the group what they wanted to be when they grew up. Thank all trainees who shared. If any trainees indicated a profession other than being a supervisor of support staff (which is likely), then point that out. Then ask all trainees who, when they thought about what they wanted to be when they grew up, wanted to do exactly what they do now for a living. Most trainees probably will not have identified working as a supervisor of support staff as a goal when they were growing up. Point out that most people who end up being supervisors did not expect to be in that profession. Then indicate an offshoot of that fact: Most people were not formally trained to be supervisors (e.g., they did not study in school how to supervise the performance of support staff). Last, make the point that the lack of opportunities to receive formal training on how to supervise is the reason for this training session: to present tried and tested ways to effectively supervise the performance of support staff.

The first step in effectively supervising the work performance of the staff is to know what constitutes *supervision*.

QUESTION TRAINEES

Ask trainees to think about the duties that they spend most of their time doing as part of their jobs as supervisors. Prompt several different trainees for responses to obtain a variety of job duties.

As the examples illustrate, people who work as supervisors have many duties. However, from the point of view of assisting the staff in working in a way that provides the best supports and services possible for agency clients, the job of a supervisor is quite straightforward.

SHOW SLIDE 1.1 ▶

Slide 1.1: Essence of a Supervisor's Job

The essence of a supervisor's job is two-fold. First, when staff performance is less than adequate, the job is to take action to change and improve that performance. Second, when staff performance is adequate, the job is to take action to support or reinforce that performance.

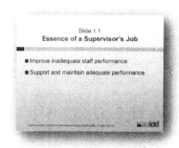

Most people agree about the first part of supervision—the importance of working to improve the performance of a staff member that is less than adequate. For example, most supervisors realize that action must be taken to change negative interactions between a staff member and an agency client, to reduce staff absenteeism, or to resolve a staff member's failure to complete work duties. In contrast, it is often less apparent that supervision also means actively working to support ongoing, adequate staff performance.

SHOW SLIDE 1.2 ▶

Slide 1.2: Importance of Supporting Good Performance of Staff

It is important to actively support good staff performance for two reasons: First, positively supporting good performance can help motivate the staff to continue performing in a quality manner; and second, supporting good staff performance helps staff members enjoy their work. The benefits of providing an enjoyable quality of work life for the staff will be discussed in depth during this training session. Conversely, there are likely to be problems when staff members *do not* enjoy their work.

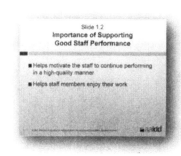

? QUESTION TRAINEES

Ask trainees about some of the problems they think result when staff members do not enjoy their work. Prompt the trainees to discuss why supervisors should be concerned about staff members' enjoyment of their work.

SHOW SLIDE 1.3 ▶

Slide 1.3: Primary Goal of This Training Session

The goal of this training session is based on the essence of supervision and the importance of providing an enjoyable work environment for the staff. Specifically, the goal is to equip supervisors with knowledge and skills to improve staff performance that needs improvement, support and maintain good performance, and help staff members enjoy their work.

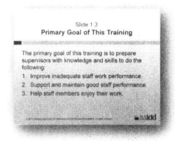

INTRODUCE EVIDENCE-BASED SUPERVISION

Evidence-Based Supervision

Before focusing on how to supervise effectively, the basis for the information to be presented warrants mention. We will be presenting *evidence-based* strategies for supervising the performance of support staff. Evidence-based supervision means the strategies have been researched and evaluated in human service settings. The research has provided evidence that the strategies, when appropriately and consistently carried out, are usually effective.

SHOW SLIDE 1.4

Slide 1.4: Importance of an Evidence-Based Approach to Supervision

Using supervisory strategies that have an evidence base to support their effectiveness is important for a variety of reasons. In particular, if supervisory approaches are relied on that do not have an established evidence base, then supervision becomes little more than guesswork. Sometimes the guesses might help to achieve the goals of supervision, but usually they will not.

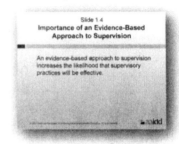

Without opportunities to receive training in evidence-based supervisory strategies, supervisors have little choice but to rely on other ways to supervise. For example, supervisors are often exposed to popular fads and traditional clichés about how to supervise. Have you ever heard advice such as "walk softly but carry a big stick" or "supervisors should be leaders"?

Such information can be appealing. However, clichés rarely are specific enough to help a supervisor know what to do in actual situations to impact staff performance or work enjoyment. Even if clichés provide some specific information, there is usually little if any sound evidence to ensure the resulting supervisory practices will be effective.

Again, this training focuses on those ways to supervise that have been shown through research and application to effectively impact staff performance and help staff members enjoy their work.

Slide 1.1
Essence of a Supervisor's Job

- Improve inadequate staff performance
- Support and maintain adequate performance

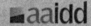

Slide 1.2
Importance of Supporting Good Staff Performance

- Helps motivate the staff to continue performing in a high-quality manner
- Helps staff members enjoy their work

Slide 1.3
Primary Goal of This Training

The primary goal of this training is to prepare supervisors with knowledge and skills to do the following:

1. Improve inadequate staff work performance.
2. Support and maintain good staff performance.
3. Help staff members enjoy their work.

Slide 1.4
Importance of an Evidence-Based Approach to Supervision

An evidence-based approach to supervision increases the likelihood that supervisory practices will be effective.

MODULE 2

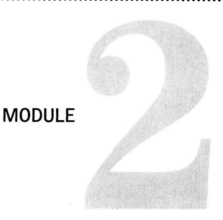

Making Performance Expectations Clear
Specifying Work Duties

The following will be covered on day 1 of training.

Objectives

Upon completion of this module, trainees should be able to do the following:

1. Describe the importance of specifying performance expectations.
2. Identify four guidelines for specifying performance expectations.
3. Identify examples of performance expectations that are and are not clearly specified.

Method

1. Presentation on importance of specifying performance expectations: *5 minutes*
2. Presentation on first two guidelines for specifying performance expectations: *5 minutes*
3. Trainer role play and trainee discussion: *10 minutes*
4. Presentation on last two guidelines for specifying performance expectations: *5 minutes*
5. Trainer presentation and trainee activity on identifying expectations that are and are not clearly specified: *10 minutes*
6. Competency check: *10 minutes*

Competency Check, Materials, and Total Training Time

1. Competency check: Completion of Competency Check Form 2.1
2. Materials
   a. PowerPoint presentation equipment (LCD, computer, curriculum CD) or

> b. Overhead projector and copies of Slides 2.1 and 2.2
>
> c. Two magazines for role play
>
> d. Competency Check Form 2.1
>
> 3. Total training time: *45 minutes*

Making Performance Expectations Clear: Specifying Work Duties

IMPORTANCE OF SPECIFYING WORK EXPECTATIONS

A critical part of supervision is making sure performance expectations are clear to the staff members. Staff members cannot be expected to do a good job if they do not know exactly what they are supposed to do on a day-to-day basis. In turn, supervisors cannot work with staff members effectively if they are not clear on precisely what staff members should be doing.

The importance of making performance expectations clear may seem readily apparent. In common practice though, job expectations, as well as work problems of concern, often are not expressed clearly. For example, have you ever heard that a staff member does not have a good work ethic? Having (or lacking) a good work ethic can mean different things.

To some people, a poor work ethic means a staff member does not show up for work consistently. To others, a poor work ethic means a staff member rarely does what is expected unless the supervisor is present. To supervise in a manner that overcomes a poor work ethic, the things that are actually *done* on the job that reflect a good versus a poor work ethic must be specified.

We will talk about other examples of how performance expectations are often presented in ways that do not make it clear what staff members should actually do on the job and problems that result for supervisors. The concern here is to recognize that to effectively supervise staff members' performance, supervisors must make sure performance expectations are very clear to staff members.

SHOW SLIDE 2.1

Slide 2.1: Guidelines for Ensuring Performance Expectations Are Clear

DESCRIBE FIRST GUIDELINE

There are four guidelines for ensuring a performance expectation is presented in a way that is clear to staff members. The first guideline is that an expectation must be described in terms of the specific *work behavior* expected of staff members. Behavior in this context refers to what a staff member does on the job. Writing a progress note, telling a client how to complete a household chore, and sweeping the porch at a group home exemplify different types of work behaviors because they refer to what a staff member is doing.

QUESTION TRAINEES

Ask several trainees to give some examples of staff members' work behaviors they expect to observe on the job. For those examples that denote specific work behaviors, tell the trainees that those are good examples of staff members' *behavior*. Be sure to politely correct any examples that do not describe behavior (e.g., inform how the examples could be more specific to indicate actual work behavior).

DESCRIBE SECOND GUIDELINE

The second guideline for ensuring a performance expectation is expressed clearly is that work behavior necessary to fulfill the expectation is described in a way that allows the behavior to be readily *observed*. Observed means what the staff member is expected to do (or not do) can be seen or, in some cases, heard. To illustrate, we can easily see if a staff member is writing a progress note or sweeping the porch, and we can hear if the staff member is speaking to a client about how to do a chore.

Consider the reference earlier regarding a work ethic. We cannot observe a "work ethic" per se. However, we can observe certain behaviors that represent a good work ethic. We can observe, for example, if a staff member always reports to work for a scheduled work shift or starts to complete job duties without a supervisor specifically telling the staff person to do each duty. We can also observe if, when a specific task is assigned by a supervisor, the staff member continues to work on that task until it is completed.

When performance expectations are expressed in terms of observable staff member behaviors, then we can begin to effectively supervise to ensure fulfillment of those expectations.

TRAINER ROLE PLAY

The two trainers should role-play two examples of staff members' work behavior. Imagine it is afternoon leisure–social time in a group home in which four people with profound intellectual disabilities live. Select three or four trainees at a table to play the roles of the clients as they sit around the table. Then inform the trainees that one trainer will play the role of a staff member who demonstrates a "lack of diligence" during the leisure-social activity. That trainer should sit in a chair close to the clients and not interact with the clients except for giving general instructions (e.g., "it is time to sit quietly"). Next, the other trainer should role-play a staff member who shows "diligence" during the activity. That trainer should walk around and interact with each client briefly and give at least one client a choice (e.g., show two magazines and ask which magazine the client would like to have). After the second role play, ask the trainees what behaviors were exhibited by each of the two staff members (role-played by the two trainers) that demonstrated a "lack of diligence" and "diligence," respectively. Emphasize that there were specific behaviors that led to a general reference of a lack of diligence and diligence.

General concepts such as diligence, work ethic, attitude, and so forth are of course important. However, because we often have varying ideas regarding what those concepts mean, it is necessary to specify the work behaviors that represent the general concepts. By focusing on specific behaviors to engage in at work, and perhaps what not to do, we can help staff members work in a way that reflects diligence, a good work ethic, and so forth. In contrast, if we only refer to the general concepts, then there will be confusion and disagreement about what a staff member should or should not do.

DESCRIBE THIRD GUIDELINE

We can tell that a performance expectation is clearly specified as an observable work behavior when we can *count* or *measure* that behavior. Hence, the third guideline is that a performance expectation must be presented in a way that we can count how often it occurs.

To illustrate, we can count how many clients a staff member speaks to upon first reporting to a group home to begin a work shift or how many teaching programs are carried out each day in a classroom. Speaking to clients and carrying out teaching programs are therefore examples of work behaviors that can be observed and measured.

Again, specifying performance expectations in a clear manner as work behavior that can be observed and measured is necessary to make sure the expectations are clear to staff members. Such specification is also critical for evaluating whether supervisory actions are effective or not. As will be highlighted later, effective supervision involves evaluating whether what a supervisor does has the desired impact on staff members' performance. Being able to observe and measure staff member behavior allows us to evaluate if our supervisory efforts are effective.

DESCRIBE FOURTH GUIDELINE

The final guideline for specifying a performance expectation is that two people must be able to agree when a designated work behavior occurs that represents the expectation. This is, in essence, the bottom line for deciding whether we have specified an expectation clearly or not. If two people can agree when the designated work behavior is occurring, then it is sufficiently specified. If two people cannot agree, then the expectation needs to be better specified.

SHOW SLIDE 2.2

Slide 2.2: Examples of Performance Expectations

DISCUSS EXAMPLES ON SLIDE 2.2

Review each performance expectation on Slide 2.2. After summarizing each expectation, ask trainees if the expectation is presented clearly in terms of specifying work *behavior,* being able to be *observed* and *counted,* and whether two people will likely *agree* when the behavior occurs. Inform trainees which expectations are not clearly presented because they do not meet the guidelines (the first and third examples) and which expectations are clearly presented (second and fourth examples) and explain how each of the latter meets the guidelines. For the two examples that are not clearly presented, explain how they could be changed to meet the guidelines and be more clear. To illustrate, explain how "courteous to family members" could be presented as greeting family members by their name, returning calls to family members within one day of the call, answering all questions of family members, and thanking family members for visiting. Similarly, for "showing initiative," explain how this could be more clearly presented (e.g., beginning and completing assigned work duties each day without being reminded by the supervisor, telling the supervisor when certain supplies are running low instead of waiting to tell the supervisor when there are no more supplies).

CONDUCT COMPETENCY CHECK

Conduct the competency check using Competency Check Form 2.1.

Slide 2.1
Guidelines for Making Performance Expectations Clear

1. Describe expectation in terms of specific work behavior.
2. Describe work behaviors so they can be observed.
3. Describe work behaviors so they can be counted.
4. Describe work behaviors so people can agree when they occur.

© 2011 American Association on Intellectual and Developmental Disabilities. All rights reserved.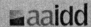

Slide 2.2
Examples of Clear and Unclear Performance Expectations

1. Always be courteous to family members of clients.
2. On the *daily time sheet,* log in your name, the time you reported for work, and time you left from work.
3. Show initiative with your work.
4. When starting a group leisure activity with clients, make sure there are at least two types of materials present so clients can choose which activity to do or how to do an activity.

© 2011 American Association on Intellectual and Developmental Disabilities. All rights reserved.

MODULE 2 COMPETENCY CHECK

Making Performance Expectations Clear: Specifying Work Duties

TRAINER INSTRUCTIONS

- Distribute Competency Check Form 2.1 to each trainee.

- Ask trainees to read each example of a performance expectation and mark "Yes" for those examples that are specified in terms of (a) behavior, (b) whether they can be observed, (c) whether they can be counted, and (d) whether two people can agree when the behavior occurs. Ask trainees to mark "No" for those examples that fail to meet at least one of the four guidelines just noted (i.e., the expectation is not specified as behavior, cannot be observed, cannot be counted, or two people would likely have difficulty agreeing when the performance occurred).

- Allow no more than 10 minutes for the activity

MASTERY CRITERION

Trainees must answer at least 4 out of 5 examples correctly.

ANSWERS

1. Yes
2. No
3. No
4. Yes
5. Yes

MODULE 2 COMPETENCY CHECK FORM 2.1

Making Performance Expectations Clear: Specifying Work Duties

Trainee name: _____ Date: _____

INSTRUCTIONS

For each of the following performance expectations, put a check mark next to "Yes" for those that are specified in terms of behaviors that can be both observed and counted and that two people would likely agree on when they occur. Put a check mark next to "No" for those that are not expressed as behaviors, could not be observed or counted, or two people would have difficulty agreeing on when they occurred.

1. Begin each teaching program that is written on the daily schedule within 15 minutes of the scheduled time for the program.

    Yes _____ No _____

2. Use appropriate language when interacting with agency clients.

    Yes _____ No _____

3. Manage use of agency equipment and materials wisely.

    Yes _____ No _____

4. When unable to report for a scheduled work shift due to illness, call immediate supervisor no later than two hours before the shift starts, and inform the supervisor of the forthcoming absence.

    Yes _____ No _____

5. When spending money from the petty cash fund, answer all questions on the Petty Cash Form (located in the house office) on the same day that the money is spent.

    Yes _____ No _____

FOR TRAINER RECORDING

Total number correctly answered: _____

Criterion met (minimum of 4 correct answers)?   Yes _____   No _____

MODULE 3

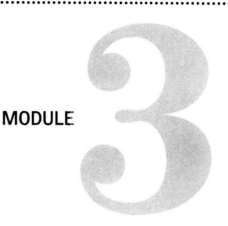

Making Performance Expectations Clear
Job Duty Checklists

The following will be covered on day 1 of training.

Objectives

Upon completion of this module, trainees should be able to do the following:

1. Describe a job duty checklist.
2. Identify when checklists are helpful.
3. Develop a job duty checklist.

Method

1. Presentation on what a checklist is and when checklists are helpful: *2 minutes*
2. Presentation on examples of checklists: *8 minutes*
3. Trainer role play and trainee activity: *15 minutes*
4. Presentation and trainee discussion on job duties for which checklists are helpful: *15 minutes*
5. Competency check: *15 minutes*

Competency Check, Materials, and Total Training Time

1. Competency check: Completion of Competency Check Form 3.1
2. Materials
   a. PowerPoint presentation equipment (LCD, computer, curriculum CD) or
   b. Overhead projector and copies of Slides 3.1, 3.2, and 3.3
   c. Activity Sheet 3.1 and sheets of paper
   d. Competency Check Form 3.1
3. Total training time: *55 minutes*

INTRODUCE CHECKLISTS

Making Performance Expectations Clear: Job Duty Checklists

In Module 2 we talked about the importance of making performance expectations very clear for the staff. We discussed that for job expectations to be clear, they should be described as specific *behaviors* that can be *counted* and easily *observed* such that two people could agree when they occur. In this session we will talk about another way to make performance expectations clear through job duty *checklists*.

Checklists describe each specific behavior that must be performed to complete a given job duty. Checklists are like task analyses of skills that we often use when teaching people with intellectual disabilities. The checklists break down job duties into specific staff member behaviors just as task analyses break down target skills for clients into specific behaviors or steps.

Checklists are especially useful when a series of behaviors must be performed in a certain order to adequately complete a job duty. Checklists are also really helpful when the job duty is rather complex in terms of requiring a large number of steps to complete.

SHOW SLIDE 3.1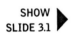

Slide 3.1: First Example of a Job Duty Checklist (Conducting a Monthly Inventory of Group Leisure Materials)

TRAINER NOTE

Note that this checklist shows just one way that the job of completing an inventory of leisure materials could be represented. Note also that each agency or supervisor must decide what the primary steps of a job duty should be and that how to develop a checklist will be discussed shortly.

This checklist specifies one way to conduct an inventory of materials used during leisure time in a group home for people with severe disabilities. The intent of the checklist is to ensure that each month a staff member checks each leisure item and informs the supervisor about items that need to be replaced because they are damaged or missing. In this manner, there will be an ongoing system for ensuring an adequate supply of leisure materials. In contrast, if there is no means of regularly checking and replacing leisure items, then at times the staff will have no materials available to promote client leisure activity.

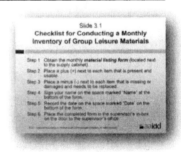

SHOW SLIDE 3.2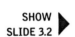

Slide 3.2: Second Example of a Job Duty Checklist (Leaving for Lunch)

This checklist provides specific information about what a staff member should do if the person leaves the work site during a lunch break.

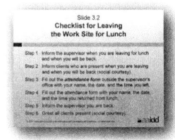

The checklist is designed to ensure staff members know what to do when leaving the work site so that appropriate staff coverage can be maintained and everyone is aware that the staff member will be gone for a period of time. It also includes several social courtesy components.

As with the checklist for conducting an inventory of leisure items, this checklist does not mean that the staff in all agencies should follow these steps when leaving for lunch. This is just an example of how it is expected to be done in one agency. Again, each agency or supervisor must decide which specific steps should go into a checklist to make sure fulfilling the job expectation is clear to the staff.

TRAINER ROLE PLAY AND TRAINEE ACTIVITY

Hand out Activity Sheet 3.1. Ask trainees to watch as one trainer prepares a client worktable for two clients to begin the work task of collating manual pages. Also, ask trainees to write each step the trainer completes on the activity sheet in the spaces marked Step 1, 2, 3, and so on. Prior to the demonstration, the trainer should remove all chairs from one table and scatter a few items on the table (e.g., a coffee cup, crumpled pieces of paper). Then for the demonstration, the trainer should do each of the following steps in order: (a) remove all items from the table, (b) wipe the table with a napkin, (c) place two chairs on one side of the table, (d) place two stacks of paper in front of one chair on the table, and (e) place two stacks of paper in front of the other chair. The trainer should then ask one trainee to share which steps she or he listed on the activity sheet and encourage discussion about whether his or her listing of the steps is the same as those listed by other trainees (there is likely to be disagreement among trainees). Then repeat the demonstration slowly while describing each of the five steps.

The process we just went through illustrates how to make a job duty checklist. There are two ways to do this. One way is to watch as someone does the duty and write down each of the key behaviors necessary to complete the duty. The second way is to do the task yourself and write down each behavioral step as you do it. When the first way is used, it is a good idea to then do the duty yourself and check to make sure you have the steps listed in the right way.

The most important thing when developing a checklist is to have the behavioral steps listed in the specific way you want the staff to perform the duty. To be clear to the staff, each step in the checklist must specify behavior, be observable, be countable or measurable, and be described such that two people would likely agree when the step is completed.

SHOW SLIDE 3.3

Slide 3.3: Examples of Job Duties Often Specified With a Checklist for the Staff

As noted earlier, checklists are especially helpful for job duties that are complex because they involve a number of specific actions to complete.

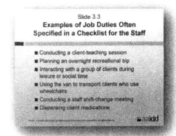

MODULE 3: MAKING PERFORMANCE EXPECTATIONS CLEAR | 25

This slide shows examples of job duties that are often specified with a checklist to help make sure staff members know what to do to complete the duties.

QUESTION TRAINEES

Ask several trainees to name some job duties that they use checklists for or for which they think checklists would be helpful for the staff.

REFER TO ON-THE-JOB TRAINING

One of the things we will look for when we come to your work site for the on-the-job portion of this training is a checklist that you have developed for your staff. We will talk more about this part of the training later. At this point, it would just be helpful to be thinking about a job duty for which you could develop a checklist.

PRACTICAL QUALIFICATION WITH CHECKLISTS

One final point about checklists and specifying performance expectations in general: It is unrealistic to specify every job expectation of the staff in the ways we have been discussing. Generally, though, as many performance expectations as possible should be specified. Certainly, those expectations that are the most important for agency staff to fulfill should be carefully specified.

Duties that pertain to serious health issues of clients, for example, are always very important. To illustrate, if a client who has a history of eating dangerous items lives in a group home, then a checklist should be available to the staff to make it clear how to maintain a safe environment (e.g., routinely checking the home to remove small items accessible to a client to ingest, making sure dangerous cleaning fluids are in a locked container).

Any performance area that is causing significant problems for the staff should also be carefully specified. For example, if there are problems with clients showing up at a day program without necessary items such as an individual's eyeglasses or a person's communication device, then a checklist should be available to the staff to help check the presence of the items before the clients leave the home to go to the day program.

CONDUCT COMPETENCY CHECK

Hand out Competency Check Form 3.1. Review the instructions at the top of the form. As each group of trainees is finishing the process, circulate among the groups and review each trainee's checklist. If necessary, work with respective trainees until a satisfactory checklist is completed in that each step specifies behavior that can be observed, counted, and two people would likely agree if each step occurred or not. Collect the forms from each trainee.

Slide 3.1
Checklist for Conducting a Monthly Inventory of Group Leisure Materials

Step 1   Obtain the monthly *material listing form* (located next to the supply cabinet).

Step 2   Place a plus (+) next to each item that is present and usable.

Step 3   Place a minus (-) next to each item that is missing or damaged and needs to be replaced.

Step 4   Sign your name on the space marked "Name" at the bottom of the form.

Step 5   Record the date on the space marked "Date" on the bottom of the form.

Step 6   Place the completed form in the supervisor's in-box on the door to the supervisor's office.

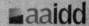

© 2011 American Association on Intellectual and Developmental Disabilities. All rights reserved.

Slide 3.2
Checklist for Leaving the Work Site for Lunch

Step 1   Inform the supervisor when you are leaving for lunch and when you will be back.

Step 2   Inform clients who are present when you are leaving and when you will be back (social courtesy).

Step 3   Fill out the *attendance form* outside the supervisor's office with your name, the date, and the time you left.

Step 4   Fill out the attendance form with your name, the date, and the time you returned from lunch.

Step 5   Inform the supervisor you are back.

Step 6   Greet all clients present (social courtesy).

© 2011 American Association on Intellectual and Developmental Disabilities. All rights reserved.

Slide 3.3
Examples of Job Duties Often Specified in a Checklist for the Staff

- Conducting a client-teaching session
- Planning an overnight recreational trip
- Interacting with a group of clients during leisure or social time
- Using the van to transport clients who use wheelchairs
- Conducting a staff shift-change meeting
- Dispensing client medications

MODULE 3 ACTIVITY SHEET 3.1

Making Performance Expectations Clear: Job Duty Checklists

Trainee name: _____ Date: _____

INSTRUCTIONS

As the trainer prepares the worktable, list each step (trainer action) below that the trainer performs.

CHECKLIST FOR PREPARING A WORKTABLE FOR TWO CLIENTS TO COLLATE MANUAL PAGES

Step	Trainer Action
1	_____
2	_____
3	_____
4	_____
5	_____

MODULE 3 COMPETENCY CHECK

Making Performance Expectations Clear: Job Duty Checklists

TRAINER INSTRUCTIONS

- Distribute Competency Check Form 3.1 to each trainee.
- Read the instructions at the top of the form to the group of trainees.
- Instruct the trainees to read the instructions themselves and complete the activity.
- Allow no more than 20 minutes for the activity.

MASTERY CRITERION

Each trainee must list action steps on Competency Check Form 3.1 in a manner that specifies behavior, can be observed, can be counted or measured, and is written such that two people would likely agree when it occurs.

MODULE 3 COMPETENCY CHECK FORM 3.1

Making Performance Expectations Clear: Job Duty Checklists

Trainee name: _____ Date: _____

INSTRUCTIONS

Some staff members are not appropriately notifying a work site when they will be late reporting for their work shifts (e.g., because their cars will not start). To ensure the work site supervisor will know a staff member will be late, a checklist needs to be developed for informing staff members how to notify the supervisor when they will be late. As a group, develop a checklist that specifies what a staff member should do when it is likely she or he will be late (e.g., whom to call, what information to provide). Determine the actions that are relevant to your work site (there will be some actions that are probably relevant for work sites of all trainees in your group and some that are specific to your work site). Each trainee should share his or her completed checklist with the other trainees who then should determine if the checklist is specific enough so that he or she would know the procedure for calling in at the trainee's work site.

CHECKLIST FOR CALLING IN LATE AT A WORK SITE

Step	Specific Action
1	_____
2	_____
3	_____
4	_____
5	_____
6	_____
7	_____

MODULE 4

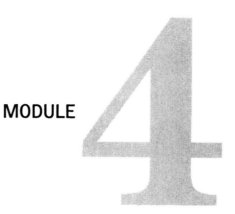

Assessing Work Performance
Formal Monitoring

The following will be covered on day 1 of training.

Objectives

Upon completion of this module, trainees should be able to do the following:

1. Identify the purposes of monitoring in supervision.
2. Observe staff work performance with a checklist.
3. Observe staff performance by counting work behavior.
4. Observe the products of staff work performance with a checklist.

Method

1. Presentation on evidence-based supervision and monitoring: *7 minutes*
2. Trainer role play and trainee activity on monitoring with a checklist: *10 minutes*
3. Presentation on monitoring by counting work behavior: *3 minutes*
4. Trainer role play and trainee activity on counting work behavior: *10 minutes*
5. Presentation and trainee discussion on how to use results of monitoring: *10 minutes*
6. Presentation and trainee discussion on monitoring work products: *10 minutes*
7. Presentation and trainee activity on key points for successful monitoring: *20 minutes*

> Competency Check, Materials, and Total Training Time
> 1. Competency check: To be completed during on-the-job training
> 2. Materials
>   a. PowerPoint presentation equipment (LCD, computer, curriculum CD) or
>   b. Overhead projector and copies of Slides 4.1, 4.2, 4.3, 4.4, 4.5, and 4.6
>   c. Activity Sheets 4.1 and 4.2
>   d. Bottle of soda and cup
> 3. Total training time: *1 hour and 10 minutes*

Assessing Work Performance: Formal Monitoring

REVIEW EVIDENCE-BASED SUPERVISION

As discussed earlier, the approach to supervision covered in this training is evidence based. Applied research has provided a considerable amount of evidence to support the effectiveness of the supervisory strategies we have been talking about.

There is also another type of evidence beyond supportive research that is critical to successful supervision. Supervisors themselves should obtain evidence that what they do to impact staff performance is effective. Supervisors should have *ongoing* evidence that their supervisory strategies are having the desired effect on staff behavior.

INTRODUCE MONITORING

The only way to truly know if efforts to impact staff performance are effective is to routinely *monitor* it. Monitoring involves observing staff work activity to assess the quality of their job performance. Monitoring serves two purposes that are keys to successful supervision.

SHOW SLIDE 4.1

Slide 4.1: Purpose of Monitoring Staff Work Performance

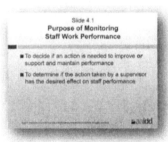

PURPOSE OF MONITORING

The first purpose is to assess staff performance so a supervisor can decide if action needs to be taken to improve the performance or to support and maintain the performance. Action is needed to improve performance if observations reveal work behavior is less than adequate. Action is needed to support the performance if observations indicate work behavior is of the desired quality.

The second purpose of monitoring is to evaluate the effects of whatever action a supervisor takes. If action is taken to improve staff performance, then results of the monitoring are used to assess if improvement results. If action is taken to support performance, then results of the monitoring are used to assess if staff members continue performing in the desired manner.

SHOW SLIDE 4.2

Slide 4.2: Three Types of Monitoring in Supervision

There are three general types of monitoring in supervision. The first type is *formal monitoring*, which we will discuss in this module. The second type is *informal monitoring*, which will be discussed in Module 5. The third type, which can accompany both formal and informal monitoring, pertains to assessing staff members' enjoyment of their work. This type will be discussed in later modules.

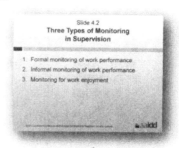

Formal monitoring can be accomplished by directly observing staff work *performance* and by observing the *product* or outcome of staff work efforts. We will focus on performance monitoring first.

Monitoring Work Performance

One of the easiest ways to monitor staff work performance is by using job duty checklists that were discussed in Module 3. Actually, one of the most important features of having checklists of staff work duties is that the checklists facilitate monitoring by a supervisor.

MONITORING WITH CHECKLISTS

TRAINEE ACTIVITY AND TRAINER ROLE PLAY

Hand out two copies of Activity Sheet 4.1 to each trainee. Read the instructions at the top of the activity sheet. Next, one trainer should slowly perform the task (same task as in Module 3—preparing a worktable for two clients to collate manual pages) and omit Step 2 (i.e., the trainer should not wipe the table). As the trainer performs the task, the other trainer should describe for the trainees what should be recorded on the activity sheet and why (i.e., a plus [+] should be marked for Steps 1, 3, 4, and 5 because the trainer completed each of those steps and a minus [–] for Step 2 because the trainer did not complete that step). Then repeat the demonstration with the trainees monitoring and scoring the second copy of the activity sheet. With the second demonstration, the trainer should correctly complete each step. The other trainer should praise the trainer's correct completion of the task when finished and then review the trainees' recordings as a group to ensure they correctly scored the checklist. Any questions that arise should also be answered.

IMPORTANCE OF PRAISE

This activity shows how a checklist can be used to observe a staff member's work performance and assess whether the staff member correctly completed the task or not. Notice also that praise was provided for correctly completing the task. Praising work performance is critical for helping staff members do a good job and enjoy their work. We will talk much more about the importance of supervisor praise later.

REFERENCE ON-THE-JOB TRAINING

In Module 3, we asked you to think about a checklist that you can develop for a staff work duty that we will want to see during the on-the-job part of

MODULE 4: ASSESSING WORK PERFORMANCE

the training. We will also want to watch as you observe a staff member perform a job duty in conjunction with the checklist you developed. Again, we will talk more about the on-the-job training later.

MONITORING BY COUNTING BEHAVIOR

Another common way to monitor staff performance is by counting how often a desired work behavior occurs. This is one reason it is important to clearly specify performance expectations in terms of behaviors that can be counted.

When formally monitoring staff performance by counting how often a work behavior occurs, it is helpful to have a prepared monitoring sheet or observation form. Consider, for example, a situation in which one staff member is assigned to be with an individual who has autism. A primary job expectation of the 1:1 staff person is to teach the individual useful skills to function as independently as possible during the daily routine. An observation form could be developed to monitor how often the staff member provides instruction during periods of the day versus doing things for the individual.

SHOW SLIDE 4.3 ▶

Slide 4.3: Monitoring Form for Teaching During the Daily Routine

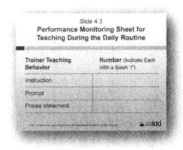

This monitoring form is designed to count a staff member's teaching behavior with the individual for whom the staff person provides 1:1 support. In this situation, teaching means the staff member provides *instruction* during the daily routine, follows the instruction with *prompting* support if the individual needs help to perform the task, and then *praises* the individual's completion of the task. The monitoring form is designed for recording how many *instructions*, *prompts*, and *praise* statements the staff member provides during a set time period (e.g., during a 15-minute work break).

TRAINEE ACTIVITY AND TRAINER ROLE PLAY

Hand out two copies of Activity Sheet 4.2 to each trainee. Review the instructions on the sheet. One trainer should then role-play the staff member being observed and the other trainer should role-play the client who has autism. Imagine the individual is at work and it is break time. The staff member is helping the individual to have a drink. The staff member should (a) present a bottle of soda and cup to the client and instruct the client to open the bottle, (b) provide a prompt by gesturing how to take the top off while telling the client how to take the top off (the client should not begin to take the top off the soda bottle following the initial instruction to open the bottle but rather should respond to the staff member's prompt), (c) praise the client's behavior after the client takes the top off, and (d) repeat the instruction, prompt, and praise sequence for helping the client pour the drink. The trainer should then describe that trainees should have recorded on the monitoring form the occurrence of 2 instructions, 2 prompts, and 2 praise statements (1 each for opening the bottle and pouring the drink). Next, instruct the trainees to use the second copy of Activity Sheet 4.2 to observe again. The trainers should repeat the role play, only this time, the trainer playing the staff member role should provide no instructions, prompts, or praise statements (the trainer should open the bottle and pour the drink for the client).

This time, your monitoring form should have zero recordings for instructions, prompts, and praise statements. Think about what the two monitoring forms show. For the first demonstration, the staff member incorporated teaching into the break routine with the client by instructing, prompting, and praising. For the second demonstration, the staff member did not include teaching into the break routine.

QUESTION TRAINEES

Ask trainees for which demonstration the monitoring suggests supervisor action is needed to change staff work behavior if we wanted the staff member to incorporate teaching into the client's break routine. Prompt trainees to discuss the second demonstration, which showed a lack of teaching behavior by the staff member. Then ask trainees which demonstration suggests, based on the monitoring, that supervisor action should be taken to support the staff member's work behavior because the staff member is doing a nice job of incorporating teaching into the break routine (i.e., the first demonstration).

See how we can use monitoring to formally assess the quality of staff teaching behavior? The monitoring provides a basis for critical decision making in supervision: deciding whether to take action to improve staff performance or to support and maintain staff performance.

In the situation just illustrated, we could continue to monitor the staff member's teaching behavior across days and see if whatever supervisory action was taken was effective in, for example, improving the behavior. If the supervisor action was effective, then we would see more instructions, prompts, and praise statements by the staff member over successive monitoring sessions. If we did not see more teaching behavior, then the supervisory action was not effective and other action would need to be taken. We will discuss actions supervisors can take to improve staff work behavior later.

The point of concern here is that to effectively supervise, and have an evidence base to show that our supervision is effective, we need to carefully monitor staff performance. We can use checklists and monitoring forms to objectively assess the quality of staff work performance and, correspondingly, the effectiveness of supervision.

Monitoring Work Products

MONITORING WORK PRODUCTS

Sometimes it is not necessary to monitor staff performance per se because the *product* or outcome of staff work activity can be monitored. Monitoring the products of staff work is often easier compared to monitoring performance because the supervisor does not have to be physically present while staff members perform the work. The supervisor can assess the quality of what staff completed at a time that fits with the supervisor's schedule.

SHOW SLIDE 4.4

Slide 4.4: Examples of Products of Staff Work Commonly Monitored by Supervisors

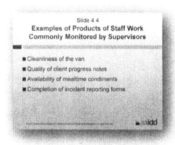

Some common products of staff work that are monitored include the cleanliness of the agency van that staff members are responsible for cleaning after community outings, the quality of client progress notes written by staff members, the availability of condiments for client choice during meal times, and accurate completion of incident reporting forms following injuries or accidents.

QUESTION TRAINEES

Ask trainees to give examples of some of the products of staff work performance that they monitor or could monitor. If necessary, elaborate on the examples to make sure they represent products or outcomes of staff performance.

WAYS TO MONITOR WORK PRODUCTS

In some cases, monitoring the product of staff work activity is as simple as recording whether a duty was completed or not within a designated time frame. In this case, records of the monitoring are just maintained to track whether staff members completed their duties on time. Examples include whether all the outside doors to a group home are locked when the clients have gone to bed or if all clients and staff have their seat belts secured prior to leaving the home in a vehicle.

In many cases though, monitoring the products of staff performance are more involved than simply checking to see if something was done on time. Often it is important to know not only if something was done but how well was it done. In these cases, for which several aspects of the product of staff work need to be monitored, monitoring is facilitated with a checklist. Instead of monitoring actual performance with a checklist as we practiced earlier, a checklist is used to monitor the quality of the product of staff performance.

SHOW SLIDE 4.4 AGAIN

Slide 4.4: Examples of Products of Staff Work Commonly Monitored by Supervisors

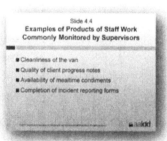

We could develop a checklist for each of these outcomes just as we developed checklists for monitoring staff performance. For example, we could develop a checklist for checking the cleanliness of the van after staff and clients return from an outing, or we could develop a checklist for evaluating if all necessary components of a progress note are in place.

PROBLEMS WITH MONITORING

Key Points for Successful Monitoring

Throughout this class session, we have noted the importance of monitoring in the overall process of supervision. It should also be acknowledged that monitoring staff performance can present some problems. These problems are not inherent in monitoring per se, but how or why staff performance is sometimes monitored.

TRAINEE ACTIVITY

Divide trainees into groups at their tables. Instruct the trainees to discuss, based on their work experience, some of the advantages and disadvantages they have seen associated with performance monitoring. Inform trainees they can refer to the experience of having their own performance monitored, of monitoring the performance of staff themselves, or of observing as other people monitor staff performance. Next, instruct the groups to reach a consensus regarding the most beneficial advantage they have experienced with monitoring *and* the biggest disadvantage or problem they have experienced with monitoring. Subsequently, ask representatives from different groups to share each consensus with the class.

SHOW SLIDE 4.5

Slide 4.5: Key Points for Avoiding Problems When Monitoring Staff Performance

Review the key points on Slide 4.5 as described below. Where relevant, relate the points to information just provided by the trainees (e.g., some of the points may have been referred to during the class discussion).

KEEP MONITORING SIMPLE

These points pertain to avoiding common problems with monitoring. The first point, *keep it simple*, means that the monitoring form or checklist should be specific and brief. Often monitoring forms are designed to gather too much information and they require substantial amounts of time to complete. When this happens, some monitors tend to do the monitoring in an incomplete manner to save time. Other monitors do not fully understand the monitoring tool and use their subjective opinion about what to record. Both of these approaches defeat the purpose of monitoring because accurate information about staff performance is not likely to result. Try to focus monitoring on the most important staff behavior during each situation and limit the amount of information to be obtained.

ONLY COLLECT INFORMATION THAT WILL BE USED

The second point, *collect only information that will be used*, pertains to a common problem in many settings. A lot of agencies collect information through monitoring that is never used to affect agency operations. The information is collected and then essentially filed.

Remember, monitoring is conducted to obtain information so a supervisor can decide to take action to improve and support staff work activity or determine if a supervisor's action impacted staff performance in the desired manner. If information collected with monitoring is not used for one of these purposes, then the monitoring probably should not be done.

The final point, *conduct monitoring in a way that is acceptable to staff*, relates to the most pervasive disadvantage of performance monitoring. Simply put, most people do not like to have their performance monitored. Supervisors need to be aware that monitoring is a part of supervision that many staff members do not like, and special effort is needed to conduct monitoring in a way that is acceptable to staff.

Fortunately, there are evidence-based means for conducting monitoring in ways that staff usually find acceptable (or at least reduces dislike of monitoring).

Slide 4.6: Steps for Making Monitoring Acceptable to Staff

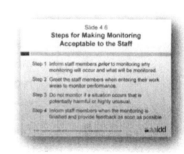

The first step for making monitoring acceptable is to make sure staff members are aware that it is part of the supervisor's job to observe their performance. Staff should also be informed before monitoring is conducted as to which aspect of their performance will be monitored. This step helps reduce potential apprehension staff may have about monitoring. It also helps reduce anxiety that can occur when staff know their performance is being monitored but do not know exactly what is being monitored.

The second step is one of social courtesy. It is common courtesy when entering a room or area in which people are present to greet the people. A supervisor should likewise greet staff when entering their work area for the specific purpose of monitoring their performance.

The third step pertains to when monitoring should be postponed. If a supervisor enters staff members' work area and a potentially harmful situation is apparent, such as a client disruptive or aggressive episode, then the supervisor should postpone the monitoring. In this type of situation, the monitor should usually help staff or otherwise find a way to resolve the situation.

Similarly, if there is a highly unusual situation when a supervisor enters staff members' work area, then monitoring generally should be postponed. This is especially the case if the situation may be potentially embarrassing to a staff member or client.

The fourth step pertains to when the monitoring is complete. As a social courtesy, the supervisor should say something to staff to indicate that he or she is leaving in contrast to simply leaving without acknowledging staff.

Additionally, it is most helpful if the supervisor provides some feedback to staff about the outcome of the monitoring. How to provide feedback will be discussed later. The point here is that staff may be somewhat anxious about how their performance was viewed. Providing feedback as soon as possible after monitoring can reduce or eliminate that anxiety.

Slide 4.1
Purpose of Monitoring Staff Work Performance

- To decide if an action is needed to improve *or* support and maintain performance
- To determine if the action taken by a supervisor has the desired effect on staff performance

Slide 4.2
Three Types of Monitoring in Supervision

1. Formal monitoring of work performance
2. Informal monitoring of work performance
3. Monitoring for work enjoyment

Slide 4.3
Performance Monitoring Sheet for Teaching During the Daily Routine

Trainer Teaching Behavior	Number (Indicate Each With a Slash "/")
Instruction	
Prompt	
Praise statement	

Slide 4.4
Examples of Products of Staff Work Commonly Monitored by Supervisors

- Cleanliness of the van
- Quality of client progress notes
- Availability of mealtime condiments
- Completion of incident reporting forms

Slide 4.5
Key Points for Avoiding Problems When Monitoring Staff Performance

1. Keep it simple.
2. Only collect information that will be used.
3. Conduct monitoring in a way that is acceptable to staff members.

Slide 4.6
Steps for Making Monitoring Acceptable to the Staff

Step 1 Inform staff members *prior* to monitoring why monitoring will occur and what will be monitored.

Step 2 Greet the staff members when entering their work areas to monitor performance.

Step 3 Do not monitor if a situation occurs that is potentially harmful or highly unusual.

Step 4 Inform staff members when the monitoring is finished and provide feedback as soon as possible.

MODULE 4 ACTIVITY SHEET 4.1: ASSESSING WORK PERFORMANCE: FORMAL MONITORING

Performance Monitoring Sheet (Preparing a Worktable)

Trainee name: _____ Date: _____

INSTRUCTIONS

As the trainer prepares the worktable for two clients to collate manual pages, score each of the following steps with a plus (+) if the trainer performed the step or a minus (−) if the trainer did not perform the step.

Step	Trainer Action	Completed (+)/Not Completed (−)
1	Removes all items from table	_____
2	Wipes table	_____
3	Places 2 chairs on 1 side of table	_____
4	Places 2 stacks of paper in front of 1 chair	_____
5	Places 2 stacks of paper in front of other chair	_____

MODULE 4 ACTIVITY SHEET 4.2: ASSESSING WORK PERFORMANCE: FORMAL MONITORING

Performance Monitoring Sheet (For 1:1 Teaching During the Daily Routine)

Trainee name: _____ Date: _____

INSTRUCTIONS

As the trainer works with the client during break time, record a slash (/) for each instruction, prompt (following an instruction), and praise statement provided by the trainer to the client. Use the following definitions:

Instruction: A direction to the client to perform a specific behavior.

Prompt: Assistance (vocal, gestural, or physical) provided to the client to help perform a behavior specified in the initial instruction.

Praise: Approval expressed to the client for performing the instructed behavior.

Trainer Teaching Behaviors	*Number*
Instruction	_____
Prompt	_____
Praise statement	_____

MODULE 5

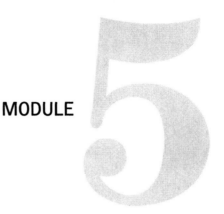

Assessing Work Performance
Informal Monitoring

The following will be covered on day 1 of training.

Objectives

Upon completion of this module, trainees should be able to do the following:

1. Identify three reasons for the importance of informal monitoring in supervision.
2. Identify three characteristics that make informal monitoring successful.
3. Demonstrate a successful example of informal monitoring.

Method

1. Presentation and trainee discussion on importance of informal monitoring: *15 minutes*
2. Presentation and trainee discussion on how to do informal monitoring: *10 minutes*
3. Trainer demonstration of informal monitoring: *10 minutes*
4. Competency check: *15 minutes*

Competency Check, Materials, and Total Training Time

1. Competency check: Completion of Competency Check Form 5.1
2. Materials
   a. PowerPoint presentation equipment (LCD, computer, curriculum CD) or
   b. Overhead projector and copies of Slides 5.1, 5.2, and 5.3
   c. Competency Check Form 5.1
3. Total training time: *50 minutes*

Assessing Work Performance: Informal Monitoring

INTRODUCE INFORMAL MONITORING

Our last session addressed the role of monitoring in an evidence-based approach to supervision. The focus was on formally monitoring staff performance using checklists and observation forms. There is also another way to monitor staff work that is just as important as formal monitoring but is usually easier to do. That way is *informal monitoring*.

Informal monitoring involves a supervisor making quick, on-the-spot observations of what staff members are doing in contrast to arranging a set time to observe with a checklist or observation form. The most common example is when a supervisor happens to be present in the staff work area and takes a minute or so to look and see what staff members are doing.

QUESTION TRAINEES

Ask trainees why it might be important for a supervisor to make quick observations of staff work behavior informally when the supervisor is present in the staff work area. Prompt several different ideas from different trainees.

SHOW SLIDE 5.1

Slide 5.1: Importance of Informal Monitoring

As the points on the overhead are reviewed with the following presentation, relate the points to reasons presented by trainees (e.g., note that some of the points may be the same as, or similar to, the points made by the trainees).

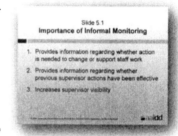

FIRST REASON OF IMPORTANCE

The first reason informal monitoring is important is the same for formal monitoring. Making quick, on-the-spot observations of ongoing staff work helps a supervisor obtain information about whether action is needed to change or support staff performance. The information is not as detailed as that obtained when monitoring formally with checklists or observation forms, but it still provides useful information about the quality of staff performance.

SECOND REASON OF IMPORTANCE

The second reason informal monitoring is important is also the same for formal monitoring. Informal monitoring helps a supervisor evaluate if previous supervisory action has had the desired effect on staff performance.

THIRD REASON OF IMPORTANCE

The third reason informal monitoring is important is that it increases supervisor *visibility*. Visibility means that the staff members often see their supervisor; the supervisor is visible to the staff. This is particularly important for supervisors who supervise staff members in a variety of different locations such that the supervisor is not continuously present in the staff work areas.

QUESTION TRAINEES

Ask trainees why supervisor visibility can be important. Make sure to relate the following points to what the trainees reported.

IMPORTANCE OF SUPERVISOR VISIBILITY

Supervisor visibility is important for several reasons. When staff members see a supervisor in their work area, it provides them with easy opportunities to ask questions or seek direction from the supervisor. Sometimes it is difficult for staff members to seek out their supervisor for these purposes if the supervisor is in a different location. In other cases, staff members are reluctant to go to a supervisor's office. By being immediately available in the staff work area, it is more likely that if staff members have questions or concerns, then they will bring these immediately to the supervisor's attention.

Another benefit of a supervisor being visible pertains to staff members' enjoyment of their work, which will be discussed in more detail later. In brief though, a common complaint of many staff members is that they rarely see their supervisor. The supervisor never seems to be around, especially if there are problems for which staff members need help from the supervisor. Consequently, the supervisor is not viewed by the staff as being very helpful. If a supervisor visits the staff work area frequently and informally monitors, then the supervisor will be very visible to staff and available to help if needed.

QUESTION TRAINEES

Ask trainees if they have experienced the opposite situation in which staff members prefer that the supervisor *not* be around very much.

In some agencies, it is common for staff members to prefer that their supervisor not be present. There are a number of reasons for this, and none of them is good. In some situations, staff members do not want their supervisor around because the supervisor frequently criticizes what staff members are doing or otherwise interacts with the staff in demeaning or unpleasant ways. In other situations, staff members are not working very hard and do not want their supervisor to see what they are doing (or not doing). The latter staff members also dislike it when they have to work harder because their supervisor is present.

These situations demonstrate another reason supervision must focus on staff work performance *and* enjoyment. These situations clearly show problems with staff performance and staff enjoyment of their work environment. Work enjoyment is impacted because the supervisor's presence represents a source of discontent for the staff. Informal monitoring, just as with other aspects of supervision, should be conducted in a way that addresses staff performance *and* adds to staff work enjoyment rather than detracting from it.

SHOW SLIDE 5.2

SUCCESSFUL WAYS TO MONITOR INFORMALLY

Slide 5.2: Characteristics of Successful Informal Monitoring

Though monitoring in the manner we have been talking about is informal, it still must be done in certain ways to promote hard work and enjoyment among the staff. For one thing, informal monitoring must have a structured basis. The supervisor must know what the staff should be doing at the time when informal monitoring occurs. When entering a staff member's work area, the supervisor should know exactly what should be going on and look to see if it is happening.

A supervisor not only should be able to tell immediately on entering a staff work site if staff members are engaging in the expected work duties but also must be able to quickly assess if staff members are performing the duties appropriately. This is another reason staff performance expectations should be specified in terms of observable work behavior.

TELL STAFF WHAT THEY ARE DOING WELL

Informal monitoring should also focus on the positive aspects of staff performance. Supervisors should always try to find what staff members are doing well and then *tell* them what they are doing well.

Letting staff members know what they are doing well involves praising or otherwise commending a specific aspect of observed performance. This action alone can go a long way in helping staff members enjoy their work.

Supervisor praise that accompanies informal monitoring also can help make the supervisor's presence in the staff work area a pleasant event for staff members. When staff members expect that a supervisor will recognize their good work, they usually like to see the supervisor in their work area.

TRAINER DEMONSTRATION

Instruct trainees that informal monitoring can be built into almost any supervisor activity that occurs in the staff work area. Then inform the trainees that if you as the trainer of this class were the trainees' supervisor, then you should be informally monitoring their performance in class. Then provide praise specific to some things you have seen a trainee or group of trainees recently do (e.g., they answered questions you have asked, they attended or looked at you while you were talking). Note that what you just did is an illustration of how to informally monitor. You as the trainer know what trainees should be doing (i.e., the things that you pointed out), you observed it happening, and then you praised some of those things.

SHOW SLIDE 5.3

Slide 5.3: Key Indicator of Good Supervision

Informal monitoring of staff performance is a critical part of effective supervision. It should be done often, and it should be accompanied by explicit approval of quality work performance as much as possible. Good supervisors continuously monitor staff performance on an informal basis, base their actions on what they observe, and frequently let staff members know when they are doing a good job.

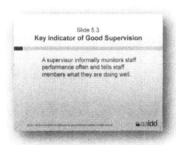

CONDUCT COMPETENCY CHECK

Conduct the competency check using Competency Check Form 5.1.

Slide 5.1
Importance of Informal Monitoring

1. Provides information regarding whether action is needed to change or support staff work

2. Provides information regarding whether previous supervisor actions have been effective

3. Increases supervisor visibility

Slide 5.2
Characteristics of Successful Informal Monitoring

1. Based on knowing what staff members should be doing at specific times

2. Based on being able to quickly tell if staff performance is adequate

3. Focused on desirable aspects of what staff members are doing and involves letting them know what they are doing well

Slide 5.3
Key Indicator of Good Supervision

A supervisor informally monitors staff performance often and tells staff members what they are doing well.

MODULE 5 COMPETENCY CHECK

Informal Monitoring

TRAINER INSTRUCTIONS

- Distribute Competency Check Form 5.1 to each trainee.//
- Read the instructions on the top of the form.
- Provide some examples of staff behavior that the supervisor may seek to observe in order to praise desirable work behavior, such as the staff member asking the client what type of a snack he or she wants, instructing the client to write the name of a snack item on the list, or praising a client's response to one of the staff member's instructions.
- Allow no more than 15 minutes for the activity.

MASTERY CRITERIA

Trainees must receive a "Yes" recording for both items indicated on the bottom of the Module 5 Competency Check Form.

MODULE 5 COMPETENCY CHECK FORM 5.1

Informal Monitoring

Trainee name: _____ Date: _____

INSTRUCTIONS

Each trainee should take a turn fulfilling each of these roles: (a) a staff member providing support to a client with intellectual disabilities who is vocal, (b) the client just referred to, and (c) a supervisor. Imagine a situation in which all three people are sitting at a table. The supervisor is making a grocery list for all clients who reside in the home. The staff member is sitting next to the client and is making a list of snack items just for the client based on the client's preferences (that the supervisor will incorporate into the master list). The desired staff performance is that while making the list, the staff member should solicit the client's opinion about snacks to put on the list and involve the client in writing the list. While working on the master list, the supervisor should informally monitor the staff member's performance and then praise at least one of the behaviors. After the role play, which should last only a few minutes, the trainee playing the role of the client should then answer the following questions about the supervisor's performance by placing a check mark in the appropriate blank.

1. Did the supervisor specify to the staff member at least one desirable work behavior that the staff member performed?

    Yes _____   No _____

2. Did the supervisor specifically praise the staff member's performance of at least one desirable work behavior by expressing approval or commendation for the behavior?

    Yes _____   No _____

FOR TRAINER RECORDING

Did the supervisor receive a "Yes" for both aspects of informal monitoring?

Yes _____   No _____

MODULE 6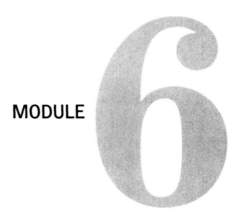

Improving and Supporting Work Performance
Diagnostic Feedback

The following will be covered on day 1 of training.

Objectives

Upon completion of this module, trainees should be able to do the following:

1. Describe the importance of supervisor feedback.
2. Describe the seven steps of diagnostic feedback.
3. Demonstrate the steps of diagnostic feedback.

Method

1. Presentation and trainee discussion on importance of giving feedback to staff: *5 minutes*
2. Presentation on steps of diagnostic feedback: *10 minutes*
3. Trainer demonstration and trainee activity on how to provide diagnostic feedback: *10 minutes*
4. Competency check: *15 minutes*
5. Presentation and trainee discussion on special considerations with feedback: *10 minutes*

Competency Check, Materials, and Total Training Time

1. Competency check
   a. Completion of Competency Check Form 6.1
   b. On-the-job demonstration of diagnostic feedback with Competency Check Form 6.1
2. Materials
   a. PowerPoint presentation equipment (LCD, computer, and curriculum CD) or

> b. Overhead projector and copies of Slides 6.1, 6.2, 6.3, and 6.4
> c. Activity Sheet 6.1
> d. Competency Check Form 6.1
> 3. Total training time: *50 minutes*

Improving and Supporting Work Performance: Diagnostic Feedback

In the last session the importance of what a supervisor should do after informally monitoring staff performance was stressed.

QUESTION TRAINEES

Ask trainees if they remember what a supervisor should do after informally monitoring staff performance. Prompt trainees to discuss the importance of telling staff members what they did well.

INTRODUCE FEEDBACK

Telling staff what they have done well represents a way of responding to staff work behavior by giving *feedback* about their performance. This session expands on how feedback should be provided to promote quality staff performance. The method for presenting feedback to be discussed also helps promote staff enjoyment of their work.

SHOW SLIDE 6.1

Slide 6.1: Importance of Feedback

Providing feedback is a critical supervisory skill. Feedback is the most readily available means through which a supervisor can improve and support staff performance *and* promote work enjoyment. Giving feedback requires no agency resources beyond a supervisor's time and effort.

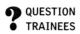

Feedback is also very effective; it impacts staff performance in many, many situations. There is more evidence to support the effectiveness of supervisor feedback than any other means of improving and supporting day-to-day staff performance.

SHOW SLIDE 6.2

Slide 6.2: Diagnostic Feedback

The most thorough way to give feedback is through *diagnostic feedback*. Diagnostic feedback involves letting staff know specifically what they did well and, if relevant, what they did not do so well. In this manner, a *diagnosis* of the proficiency of staff work performance is conducted. Diagnostic feedback also includes information about how staff can correct any performance areas that they did not do well.

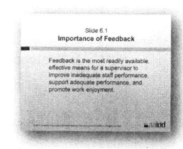

58 | THE SUPERVISOR TRAINING CURRICULUM

SHOW SLIDE 6.3

Slide 6.3: How to Give Diagnostic Feedback

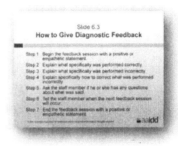

Besides being used to improve or support daily staff performance, feedback should be provided in a manner that is likely to be well received by staff. If staff members like how their supervisor gives feedback, then it can enhance enjoyment of their work situation relative to receiving feedback in a manner they do not like. The steps shown here have been demonstrated as a way to provide feedback that is usually well received by staff.

REVIEW FEEDBACK STEPS

FEEDBACK STEP 1

The first step in providing diagnostic feedback is to begin with a generally positive statement related to the staff member's work. It can be as simple as the supervisor saying that the staff person's efforts are appreciated or that it is clear the staff member is working hard. A positive statement can also be empathetic in nature (e.g., "I know that is a tough task to do").

It is important to begin the feedback session on a positive note for several reasons. Sometimes staff members become anxious when their supervisor meets with them, and beginning in a positive way can help reduce the anxiety. At other times, staff members have a history of supervisors criticizing what they do and expect the forthcoming interaction will be critical as well. When a supervisor begins the interaction with a positive comment, the staff member usually realizes the intent is not just to criticize his or her work.

FEEDBACK STEP 2

The second step of diagnostic feedback is to immediately specify those aspects of staff performance that the staff member did well. This step not only serves the same positive function as the first step but also supports the staff member in continuing to perform those job aspects in a quality fashion.

FEEDBACK STEPS 3 AND 4

The third step is to specify any aspects of performance that were not performed correctly. The fourth step is to tell exactly what the staff member should do to correct the incorrect work behavior. These two steps help staff improve work performance.

FEEDBACK STEP 5

The fifth step involves asking the staff member if there are any questions about what was said. This step helps ensure the feedback is understood. It also allows the staff member to clarify any misconceptions the supervisor may have had. For example, sometimes there are special circumstances affecting the staff person's performance, and the supervisor needs to know these to make sure the feedback is relevant to the staff member's situation.

FEEDBACK STEP 6

The sixth step involves telling the staff member when this particular performance area will be observed again and feedback will be provided. By indicating feedback will again be provided, it usually becomes clear that a supervisor considers this area of the staff member's work to be very important.

Letting staff know their performance will continue to be monitored and feedback will be provided also can motivate staff to try harder to perform

FEEDBACK STEP 7

with greater quality. Most people will try to get something right if they know that their supervisor will be coming to observe and discuss the performance.

The final step of diagnostic feedback is to end the feedback session on a positive or upbeat note, just as the feedback session began. This usually involves summarizing the positive aspects of the observed performance already commented on or simply thanking the staff member for listening. This step helps make the process of receiving feedback a pleasant experience.

TRAINER ROLE PLAY AND TRAINEE ACTIVITY

Hand out Activity Sheet 6.1 to each trainee. One trainer should play the role of a supervisor and another trainer should play the role of a staff member. Ask one of the trainees to play the role of a client who does not speak. Inform the other trainees they should watch as the supervisor gives feedback and score the supervisor's performance on the activity sheet. Read the instructions on the activity sheet. Ask the trainees to imagine that the staff member is a job coach for the client who has just been assisted in cleaning the room as part of a supported job and it is time to go clean another room. Also indicate that, due to the client's communication skills, the job coach should interact with the client by talking and gesturing. The staff member should then tell and motion for the client to follow him or her to leave the room (the client should respond to all staff instructions). Before going to the door, the job coach should walk with the client to the light switch and then tell and motion for the client to turn off the light. After the client turns off the light, the job coach should sign "thank you" but not say "thank you" to the client. (Note to trainer: To manually sign "thank you," see the instructions and diagram on Competency Check Form 7.1 in Module 7.) Next, the supervisor should give the staff member feedback following the steps on the activity sheet, making sure to note specifically what the staff member did correctly (e.g., told and motioned for the client to turn off the light) and incorrectly (i.e., not saying "thank you" while signing "thank you"). Finally, review how the recordings should have been made on the activity sheet (a "Yes" should have been scored for each of the seven feedback steps) and answer any trainee questions.

REVIEW FEEDBACK

Do you see how diagnostic feedback can both improve and support work performance? It can improve performance by informing a staff member what aspects of observed work performance were not done correctly and what specifically needs to be done to improve the performance. It can also support adequate performance by complimenting the staff member on those observed aspects of performance that were done well.

REFER TO ON-THE-JOB TRAINING

Because giving diagnostic feedback is such an important part of supervision, it is one of the skills that we will want to see you perform as part of the on-the-job portion of this training. We will talk more about on-the-job training later. Right now though, we will practice giving diagnostic feedback.

CONDUCT COMPETENCY CHECK

Conduct the competency check using Competency Check Form 6.1 (continue with the remainder of the module after the competency check).

Every supervisor should be able to give staff feedback about their performance in an effective manner. Again, using the feedback steps as just practiced is usually quite effective. However, there are also some special considerations when giving feedback.

SHOW SLIDE 6.4

Slide 6.4: Special Considerations When Giving Feedback

To impact staff work behavior to either improve or support the behavior, as well as to enhance staff acceptance of a supervisor's feedback, the feedback must be presented sincerely.

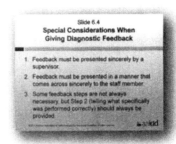

QUESTION TRAINEES

Ask trainees if they have ever been in a situation when they felt someone was complimenting their performance when they did not believe the person really knew about, or cared about, their performance. Prompt trainees to discuss how insincere feedback usually does not serve the purpose of supporting one's performance or helping one to feel good about the performance.

IMPORTANCE OF FEEDBACK BEING SINCERE

Supervisors should not tell staff they are doing a good job unless they sincerely believe the staff members are doing a good job. This is one aspect of supervision that cannot be taught in this or any other class. Each of us has to determine if we are concerned about the quality of staff performance. If we are not, then we will have difficulty giving feedback sincerely.

FEEDBACK SHOULD COME ACROSS SINCERELY

Not only does feedback have to be sincere; it has to be presented in a way that comes across to the staff as being sincere. Sometimes a supervisor is sincerely pleased after observing a staff member's performance but has difficulty expressing such pleasure in a way that appears sincere to the staff member.

For example, sometimes a supervisor works with staff members who are older and more experienced than the supervisor. In this situation, some supervisors might be nervous or feel uncomfortable telling those staff members if they are doing a good job. In other situations, supervisors simply are not very experienced at praising the activities of other adults. Fortunately, giving feedback in a way that comes across sincerely to staff is a skill that can be learned by supervisors—assuming that the supervisor is truly sincere in being pleased about staff performance.

One way to learn to present feedback in a way that comes across sincerely to staff is simply to practice giving feedback, such as by repeatedly using the feedback steps we just reviewed. Giving feedback is a performance skill, and like any other area of performance, we usually get better at it with practice.

The second way to help feedback come across sincerely is to specifically describe staff work behavior that was performed correctly. When staff members hear a supervisor describe in detail what they did well, they know the supervisor really paid attention to their work. This usually leaves staff with a more favorable impression than when a supervisor praises their performance in general without indicating knowledge of what they specifically did. Hence, the second step of diagnostic feedback of specifically telling staff members what they performed adequately is critical. This step should always be included when providing feedback.

SELECT MOST RELEVANT FEEDBACK STEPS

Another consideration when using the feedback steps we practiced is that, at times, not every step in the overall process will be needed. The feedback steps are designed primarily for those situations in which a supervisor is meeting with a staff member exclusively for the purpose of giving feedback. In this manner, the steps represent a rather formal way to provide feedback.

ALWAYS TELL SPECIFICALLY WHAT WAS DONE WELL

There are many other times during the course of a supervisor's job routine when feedback can be given to staff members in a less formal way. In these situations, which we will discuss later, not all steps of the feedback process need to be followed. Again though, Step 2 that involves letting staff know specifically what they did well should always be included as part of feedback.

Slide 6.1
Importance of Feedback

Feedback is the most readily available, effective means for a supervisor to improve inadequate staff performance, support adequate performance, and promote work enjoyment.

Slide 6.2
Diagnostic Feedback

Diagnostic feedback provides a *diagnosis* of staff work proficiency: It assesses and then informs staff members about what they did well, what they did not do so well (if relevant), and how to correct the latter.

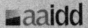

Slide 6.3
How to Give Diagnostic Feedback

Step 1 Begin the feedback session with a positive or empathetic statement.
Step 2 Explain what specifically was performed correctly.
Step 3 Explain what specifically was performed incorrectly.
Step 4 Explain specifically how to correct what was performed incorrectly.
Step 5 Ask the staff member if he or she has any questions about what was said.
Step 6 Tell the staff member when the next feedback session will occur.
Step 7 End the feedback session with a positive or empathetic statement.

© 2011 American Association on Intellectual and Developmental Disabilities. All rights reserved.

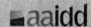

Slide 6.4
Special Considerations When Giving Diagnostic Feedback

1. Feedback must be presented sincerely by a supervisor.

2. Feedback must be presented in a manner that comes across sincerely to the staff member.

3. Some feedback steps are not always necessary, but Step 2 (telling what specifically was performed correctly) should always be provided.

© 2011 American Association on Intellectual and Developmental Disabilities. All rights reserved.

MODULE 6 ACTIVITY SHEET 6.1: DIAGNOSTIC FEEDBACK

Diagnostic Feedback Monitoring Form

Trainee name: _____ Date: _____

INSTRUCTIONS

As the supervisor gives feedback to the staff member, put a check mark next to "Yes" if the supervisor implemented the step, next to "No" if the supervisor did not implement the step, or next to "NA" (not applicable) if there was no opportunity to implement the step.

DIAGNOSTIC FEEDBACK STEPS

1. Begins the feedback session with a positive or empathetic statement:

    Yes _____ No _____

2. Specifies at least one work behavior the staff member performed correctly:

    Yes _____ No _____

3. Specifies at least one work behavior the staff member did not perform correctly (if applicable):

    Yes _____ No _____ NA _____

4. Describes how the behavior performed incorrectly should be performed (if applicable):

    Yes _____ No _____ NA _____

5. Asks the staff member if he or she has any questions, or otherwise gives the staff member an opportunity to seek clarification:

    Yes _____ No _____

6. Informs the staff member when the next feedback session will occur:

    Yes _____ No _____

7. Ends the feedback session with a positive or empathetic statement:

    Yes _____ No _____

MODULE 6 COMPETENCY CHECK

Improving and Supporting Work Performance: Diagnostic Feedback

TRAINER INSTRUCTIONS

- Distribute Competency Check Form 6.1 to each trainee.
- Read the instructions at the top of the form.
- Instruct trainees to follow the instructions on the form and perform the role play, with each trainee having the opportunity to play the role of the supervisor giving feedback.
- Inform trainees that a completed copy of Competency Check Form 6.1 should be turned in for each trainee.
- Allow no more than 15 minutes for the activity.

MASTERY CRITERION

Trainees must correctly perform at least 80% of the steps, and Step 2 must be one of the steps completed correctly.

MODULE 6 COMPETENCY CHECK FORM 6.1: IMPROVING AND SUPPORTING WORK PERFORMANCE: DIAGNOSTIC FEEDBACK

Giving Diagnostic Feedback

Trainee name: _____ Date: _____

INSTRUCTIONS

Imagine the supervisor has observed as a staff member provides an opportunity for four clients in a group home to participate in a group social-leisure activity. The following steps illustrate the staff member's desired performance with each client: (a) describe the leisure activity (e.g., playing a board game), (b) ask if the clients would like to participate, and (c) for those clients who are in their bedrooms, knock on each client's door before entering the bedroom to ask if those clients would like to participate. The supervisor has observed the staff member following each step correctly except on one occasion when the staff member did not knock on the client's door before entering the bedroom when going to ask the client if he or she wanted to participate. The supervisor should provide feedback to the staff member by following the steps on the Diagnostic Feedback Monitoring Form.

One trainee should play the staff member role and one trainee should play the supervisor role. Another trainee should observe as the supervisor gives feedback and on the Diagnostic Feedback Monitoring Form put a check mark next to "Yes" if the supervisor completed the step or next to "No" if the supervisor did not complete the step. Each trainee should play the role of the supervisor giving feedback and have the form completed by another trainee.

DIAGNOSTIC FEEDBACK MONITORING FORM

1. Begins feedback with positive or empathetic statement:

   Yes _____   No _____

2. Tells staff member at least one work behavior performed correctly:

   Yes _____   No _____

3. Tells staff member at least one work behavior performed incorrectly (if applicable):

   Yes _____   No _____   NA _____

4. Tells staff member specifically how to correct work behavior that was performed incorrectly (if applicable):

   Yes _____   No _____   NA _____

5. Asks staff member if he or she has any questions about the feedback:

   Yes _____   No _____

6. Tells staff member when the performance will be observed again and feedback will be provided:

   Yes _____   No _____

7. Ends feedback with positive or empathetic statement:

   Yes _____   No_____

FOR TRAINER RECORDING

1. Total number steps scored "Yes": _____

2. Total number steps scored "No": _____

3. Number of "Yes" ÷ (number of "Yes" + number of "No") = _____

   Did trainee receive at least 80% "Yes" recordings on #3 above and complete Step 2 correctly?
   _____

MODULE 7

Staff Training

The following will be covered on day 2 of training.

Objectives

Upon completion of this module, trainees should be able to do the following:

1. Identify three reasons why supervisors need to be able to train staff on the job.
2. Identify five steps of performance-based and competency-based staff training.
3. Demonstrate performance-based and competency-based staff training.

Method

1. Presentation and trainee discussion on importance of supervisors being able to train staff on the job: *10 minutes*
2. Presentation on performance-based and competency-based staff training: *10 minutes*
3. Trainer demonstrations and trainee activity on training staff: *20 minutes*
4. Competency check 7.1: *15 minutes*
5. Competency check 7.2: *15 minutes*

Competency Check, Materials, and Total Training Time

1. Competency check: Completion of Competency Check Forms 7.1 and 7.2
2. Materials
   a. PowerPoint presentation equipment (LCD, computer, curriculum CD) or
   b. Overhead projector and copies of Slides 7.1, 7.2, 7.3, and 7.4
   c. Activity Sheet 7.1
   d. Competency Check Forms 7.1 and 7.2
3. Total training time: *1 hour and 10 minutes*

Staff Training

INTRODUCE STAFF TRAINING

A key indicator of the quality of supports offered by a human service agency is a good staff training program. Staff cannot be expected to do a quality job if they do not have the knowledge and skills necessary to perform the job. Given that most support staff begin their jobs with little or no experience, agencies must train their staff in relevant work skills.

INTRODUCE ON-THE-JOB TRAINING

When we think about staff training, we often think about the various training programs that exist in our agencies such as orientation for new staff, training on issues related to abuse and neglect, or CPR training. These types of training are of course important. However, there is another type of training that is as important as any formal training program offered in a human service agency: the *on-the-job training* that a supervisor provides for the staff.

QUESTION TRAINEES

Ask trainees why they think it is important for a supervisor to be able to train staff. Make sure to relate their answers to the following points on Slide 7.1.

SHOW SLIDE 7.1

Slide 7.1: Why Supervisors Need to Be Able to Train Staff on the Job

IMPORTANCE OF ON-THE-JOB TRAINING

Supervisors need to be able to train staff members on the job because the other training they receive does not always carry over to their day-to-day performance. Sometimes staff members forget what they hear in orientation class as soon as they leave the class. In other cases, training that staff members receive does not relate directly to the expected tasks to be performed as part of the daily job routine.

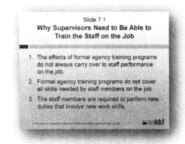

Another reason supervisors need to be able to train their staff is that it is essentially impossible for agencies to formally train all the skills that staff members need to perform their jobs. Different skills are needed depending on what part of an agency a staff member works in—such as a supported-living setting versus a day program, for example.

Supervisors also need to be able to train their staff because, over time, new duties and corresponding work skills are needed by the staff. In short, a key part of a supervisor's job is to train staff members in specific skills that are required to perform their duties appropriately.

PURPOSE OF THIS SESSION

The purpose of this session is to describe an effective means by which supervisors can train important work skills to the staff on the job. As with other strategies covered in our classes, the approach to staff training to be presented has a strong evidence base to support its effectiveness.

SHOW SLIDE 7.2

Slide 7.2: Performance-Based and Competency-Based Staff Training

The best way to train the staff in skills necessary to perform their work duties is through *performance-based* and *competency-based* training. Performance based means the training directly addresses how to perform the duties. *Competency based* means the training is not considered complete until the staff members are observed to perform the skills competently.

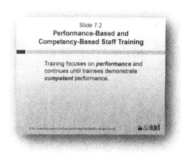

SHOW SLIDE 7.3

STEPS OF PERFORMANCE-BASED AND COMPETENCY-BASED TRAINING

Slide 7.3: Steps of Performance-Based and Competency-Based Staff Training

Performance-based and competency-based staff training involves the following steps for a supervisor. First, explain to the staff what specifically must be done to perform the duty of concern. Second, provide staff members with a written summary of the specific things they need to do.

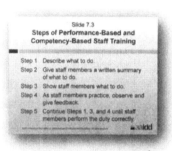

Often, a checklist of the behaviors to perform the duty, like those we discussed previously, is the best way to provide a written summary.

CONTINUE TRAINING STEPS

For example, if we wanted to train staff members to safely lift and transfer a client from a wheelchair to the bed, then we should tell the staff members how to do this and provide a checklist that specifies what to do (e.g., make sure the wheelchair is properly positioned next to the bed, lock the wheels on the wheelchair, and position one's legs about shoulder width apart to provide a good base).

The third step in performance-based and competency-based training is to show the staff how to perform the behaviors constituting the duty of concern. The fourth step is to then have the staff members practice doing the duty while the supervisor watches and provides feedback.

The act of the supervisor *performing* the duty for the staff to see and then having staff *perform* the duty while the supervisor watches represents the performance-based part of the staff training approach. These two performance steps can be done as part of the actual job or in a role-play situation during training, as we have done with some of the supervisor skills in this class.

The fourth step also involves giving feedback to the staff members regarding how well they performed the duty. The feedback should be diagnostic as discussed in the previous session. Most importantly, the feedback should specify what each staff member did correctly and, if necessary, what each staff member did incorrectly. If a staff member did something incorrectly, then the feedback also involves informing and, if necessary, showing the staff member how to do those behaviors correctly.

MODULE 7: STAFF TRAINING | 71

The final step in the training process is to repeat Steps 1, 3, and 4 until each staff member performs all aspects of the duty correctly. This final step represents the *competency-based* part of the staff training process. The training is not complete until each staff member demonstrates competence in performing the target duty.

The steps just described represent how training should occur on the job. However, this is not how it always happens. Let us show how training often occurs that is not evidence, performance, or competency based.

TRAINER DEMONSTRATION AND TRAINEE DISCUSSION

One trainer should play the role of a staff member and one trainer should play the role of a supervisor whose job is to train the staff member on how to carry out a client's behavior support plan (BSP). The supervisor in the role play should very quickly describe each component on the BSP to the staff member using the BSP steps of Activity Sheet 7.1 as a guide. While the supervisor is describing the steps, the staff member should nod his or her head as if readily understanding what the supervisor is explaining. After explaining the steps, the supervisor should ask the staff member if he or she understands how to carry out the BSP. The staff member should nod his or her head to indicate that everything is understood. The supervisor should then ask the staff member to sign a sheet of paper to indicate that the training is complete. Finally, the supervisor should ask the trainees if they think the training is likely to be successful and the staff member really knows how to carry out the BSP. Prompt the trainees to discuss how we would not know for sure whether the staff member can carry out the BSP because, for example, the staff member has not been *observed* carrying out the BSP appropriately.

As indicated before the demonstration, though this process is how training is frequently performed, it is usually not effective. Now watch as we train using the performance-based and competency-based approach to staff training.

TRAINER DEMONSTRATION AND TRAINEE ACTIVITY

Hand out Activity Sheet 7.1: Observation Form for Training Staff to Carry Out a Behavior Support Plan. Review the instructions in the middle of the form. Next, a trainer should again play the role of a staff member and another trainer should play the role of the supervisor whose job is to train the staff member to carry out a client's BSP. Ask one of the trainees to play the role of the client, and while doing so, he or she should do everything that the supervisor and staff member ask him or her to do. The supervisor should then perform training for each step of the BSP using the performance-based and competency-based training steps: Explain each step (and give the staff member a copy of Activity Sheet 7.1 that has a checklist of the BSP procedures), demonstrate each step, have the staff member practice each step (the staff member should perform all BSP steps correctly except forget to praise the client's compliance), and then repeat the show-and-tell process and have the staff member practice the BSP steps (this time the staff member should perform all BSP steps correctly). Prompt trainees to discuss how each step of the performance-based and competency-based training approach was followed by the supervisor (and how they should have scored the form).

The training method we just demonstrated can be used to train staff in just about any skill necessary to perform a job duty. Again, we tell what to do, show what to do, watch as the staff members practice and give feedback, and continue to do this until we observe them perform the skill correctly.

The training can be done with groups of staff on a formal basis, such as when having a meeting to train staff how to communicate with a new client who has a unique communication device. The training can also be done informally when a supervisor observes a staff member having difficulty performing a particular job duty. The same performance-based and competency-based steps can be used in both situations.

SHOW SLIDE 7.4 ▶

Slide 7.4: A Benefit of Performance-Based Training on Staff Work Enjoyment

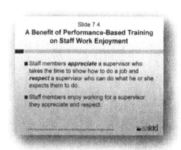

As indicated previously, this training approach has been shown many times to work effectively with support staff. There is another benefit of the training that relates to work enjoyment. Staff members usually appreciate a supervisor who takes the time to make sure they know how to do what is expected on the job.

Staff members' respect for a supervisor also increases when they see that the supervisor knows how to do what he or she expects the staff to do; this becomes evident when the supervisor demonstrates the new skill during training. Staff members usually enjoy working for a supervisor they appreciate and respect.

CONDUCT COMPETENCY CHECKS

Conduct the competency checks using Competency Check Forms 7.1 and 7.2.

Slide 7.1
Why Supervisors Need to Be Able to Train the Staff on the Job

1. The effects of formal agency training programs do not always carry over to staff performance on the job.

2. Formal agency training programs do not cover all skills needed by staff members on the job.

3. The staff members are required to perform new duties that involve new work skills.

Slide 7.2
Performance-Based and Competency-Based Staff Training

Training focuses on *performance* and continues until trainees demonstrate *competent* performance.

Slide 7.3
Steps of Performance-Based and Competency-Based Staff Training

Step 1 Describe what to do.

Step 2 Give staff members a written summary of what to do.

Step 3 Show staff members what to do.

Step 4 As staff members practice, observe and give feedback.

Step 5 Continue Steps 1, 3, and 4 until staff members perform the duty correctly.

© 2011 American Association on Intellectual and Developmental Disabilities. All rights reserved.

Slide 7.4
A Benefit of Performance-Based Training on Staff Work Enjoyment

- Staff members *appreciate* a supervisor who takes the time to show how to do a job and *respect* a supervisor who can do what he or she expects them to do.

- Staff members enjoy working for a supervisor they appreciate and respect.

© 2011 American Association on Intellectual and Developmental Disabilities. All rights reserved.

MODULE 7 ACTIVITY SHEET 7.1: STAFF TRAINING

Observation Form for Training Staff to Carry Out a Behavior Support Plan

Trainee name: _____   Date: _____

OBSERVATION FORM FOR TRAINING STAFF TO CARRY OUT A BEHAVIOR SUPPORT PLAN (BSP): CLIENT BSP PROCEDURES (STAFF TO BE TRAINED BY THE SUPERVISOR)

When the client begins to engage in repetitive finger flapping in front of her face, you should

1. walk up and face the client within 3 feet of the client;
2. calmly instruct the client to walk with you to participate in a leisure activity (e.g., go get a magazine from the shelf, turn on a DVD movie, or turn on a game on the computer);
3. praise the client when she begins to follow the instruction by walking with you.

INSTRUCTIONS

Observe as the supervisor trains the staff member to implement the BSP summarized above and put a slash (/) through the plus (+) if the supervisor implemented the training step, the minus (–) if the supervisor did not implement the step, or the "NA" (not applicable) if the supervisor did not have an opportunity to implement the step.

STAFF TRAINING STEPS

1. Describe each procedure in the BSP: +   –

2. Provide a written summary of the procedures: +   –

3. Demonstrate how to do each procedure: +   –

4. Observe as the staff trainee practiced each procedure and give feedback to the trainee: +   –

5. Repeat Steps 1, 3, and 4 until the trainee correctly performs each procedure: +   –   NA

MODULE 7 COMPETENCY CHECK 7.1

Staff Training

TRAINER INSTRUCTIONS

- Distribute Competency Check Form 7.1 to each trainee.
- Instruct the trainees to gather in small groups at their tables.
- Read the instructions on the first page of the form.
- Demonstrate how to sign "thank you" using the illustration and instructions on the form.
- Allow no more than 15 minutes for the activity.

MASTERY CRITERION

Competency Check Form 7.1 must be completed with a "Yes" recorded for each question at the bottom of the form for each trainee. (For question 5, an "NA" could also be recorded instead of "Yes" if the person being trained correctly performed the sign for "thank you" after Step 3 and a "Yes" was recorded for all other questions.)

MODULE 7 COMPETENCY CHECK FORM 7.1

Staff Training

Trainee name: _____ Date: _____

INSTRUCTIONS

Within your group, one person should play the role of the supervisor, one should play the role of the staff member being trained, and one should observe and score the form at the bottom of the page based on the supervisor's training performance. The supervisor should train the staff member how to make the manual sign for "thank you" using the illustration below as a guide and the steps of performance-based and competency-based training. The supervisor should continue training until he or she receives a "Yes" recording for each training step (an "NA" can be scored for question 5 instead of "Yes" if the trainee correctly demonstrated the sign after Step 3 and a "Yes" was recorded for all other questions). Then rotate roles until each of you has played the role of supervisor and correctly completed the training.

HOW TO SIGN "THANK YOU"

"Thank You"
With your right hand, with fingers closed and palm facing your mouth, move your hand down and out with the palm up.

Did the trainee playing the role of the supervisor do the following?

1. Explain how to make the "thank you" sign?

   Yes _____ No _____

2. Show how to do the "thank you" sign?

   Yes _____ No _____

3. Have the trainee playing the role of the staff member demonstrate the sign?

   Yes _____ No _____

4. Provide feedback to the staff member regarding his or her correctness in performing the sign?

   Yes _____ No _____

5. Repeat Steps 1–4 until the staff member correctly demonstrated how to do the "thank you" sign?

   Yes _____ No _____ NA _____

MODULE COMPETENCY CHECK 7.2

Knowledge Assessment for Modules 1 Through 7

TRAINER INSTRUCTIONS

- Distribute Competency Check Form 7.2 to each trainee.
- Instruct trainees to answer each quiz question by circling the letter next to the best answer.
- Also instruct trainees that only one answer should be circled per question.
- Allow no more than 15 minutes for the activity.

MASTERY CRITERION

Trainees must correctly answer at least 8 of the 10 questions correctly (80% correct) according to the following answer key.

ANSWER KEY

1. C
2. B
3. A
4. B
5. D
6. B
7. C
8. A
9. D
10. C

MODULE 7 COMPETENCY CHECK FORM 7.2: STAFF TRAINING

Knowledge Assessment for Modules 1 Through 7

Trainee name: _____ Date: _____

1. With respect to promoting quality work performance among support staff, the main essence of a supervisor's job is to

    A. overcome a poor work ethic among staff
    B. motivate by example
    C. change inadequate staff performance and support adequate performance
    D. instruct, monitor, and reprimand as necessary

2. Evidence-based supervision is best characterized by

    A. developing a key slogan and then supervising by following the slogan
    B. using supervisory strategies demonstrated through research and application to be effective
    C. using supervisory strategies that require the least effort yet have the biggest impact on staff performance
    D. following one's intuition about how to supervise

3. Performance expectations of staff should be presented according to that which can be

    A. stated as work behavior that can be observed, measured, and likely agreed on by two people when the behavior occurs
    B. stated in a way requiring staff initiative to fulfill them
    C. described based on a staff consensus about the best way to fulfill them
    D. stated in terms of work behavior that is likely to occur

4. A job duty checklist specifies

    A. all performance expectations expected of a staff member's job
    B. each work behavior required to complete a job duty
    C. the reasons a job duty should be completed
    D. all staff members expected to complete a job duty

5. Diagnostic feedback informs staff members

    A. what their daily duty assignments are
    B. what the source of job motivation is
    C. what they did well and what they did not so well
    D. what they did well, what they did not so well, and how to improve the latter

6. One purpose of monitoring staff work performance is to

    A. justify the importance of a supervisor's job
    B. assess staff performance to determine if action is needed to change or support the performance
    C. allow for documentation to be completed
    D. ensure the staff members are sufficiently threatened to work hard

7. Formal monitoring of staff performance is facilitated by

    A. doing it as quickly as possible
    B. doing it in a threatening manner
    C. using a job duty checklist
    D. using the agency's mission statement

8. For informal monitoring to be successful, it should be done

    A. frequently
    B. rarely
    C. only with staff who have work problems
    D. only with staff who usually do quality work

9. Evidence-based training of work skills to staff is

    A. usually not needed in human service agencies
    B. performance based and frequency based
    C. frequency based and competency based
    D. performance based and competency based

10. Showing the staff how to do a job

    A. is rarely necessary in quality human service agencies
    B. should not be expected of supervisors
    C. is a key part of evidence-based staff training
    D. is another way to describe evidence-based staff training

MODULE 8

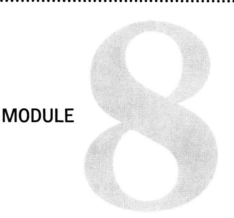

Promoting Quality Work Performance With Enjoyment

The following will be covered on day 2 of training.

Objectives

Upon completion of this module, trainees should be able to do the following:

1. Describe the importance of promoting staff work enjoyment.
2. Describe two informal ways to promote work enjoyment.
3. Describe two formal ways to promote work enjoyment.

Method

1. Presentation on review of evidence-based supervision: *5 minutes*
2. Presentation and trainee discussion on the importance of promoting staff work enjoyment: *10 minutes*
3. Presentation and trainee activity on informal ways to promote staff enjoyment of their work: *20 minutes*
4. Presentation on formal ways to promote staff enjoyment of their work: *10 minutes*
5. Competency check: *15 minutes*

Competency Check, Materials, and Total Training Time

1. Competency check: Completion of Competency Check Form 8.1
2. Materials
   a. PowerPoint presentation equipment (LCD, computer, curriculum CD) or
   b. Overhead projector and copies of Slides 8.1, 8.2, 8.3, 8.4, and 8.5
   c. Activity Sheet 8.1
   d. Competency Check Form 8.1
3. Total training time: *1 hour*

Promoting Quality Work Performance With Enjoyment

REVIEW ESSENCE OF SUPERVISOR'S JOB

We began this training session by noting that the essence of a supervisor's job is to change inadequate staff performance and to support quality performance. A number of evidence-based strategies have been presented that can help supervisors fulfill these job functions.

SHOW SLIDE 8.1

Slide 8.1: Summary of Evidence-Based Supervisory Strategies

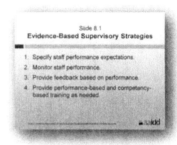

REVIEW EVIDENCE-BASED SUPERVISION

To review briefly, effective supervision begins with specifying performance expectations of staff as work behavior that can be clearly observed and measured. Staff work behavior should then be routinely monitored, both formally and informally. Monitoring in turn should be followed by supervisor feedback presented to staff. Supervisors must also be able to provide performance-based and competency-based training to ensure staff members have the skills to perform their job duties.

FOCUS NOW ON WORK ENJOYMENT

The focus in discussing these keys to effective supervision has been to promote quality staff performance. To a lesser degree, ways to use the procedures to enhance staff enjoyment of their work have also been noted. This module focuses more specifically on how to help staff members enjoy their work.

Earlier we talked a little bit about why supervisors should strive to help staff members enjoy their work. Remember when we discussed some of the problems that arise when staff members do not enjoy their work?

 QUESTION TRAINEES

Ask trainees to briefly summarize the problems they noted when staff members do not enjoy their work. If necessary, remind trainees of some of the problems they brought up in the first training session.

Sometimes supervisors question the importance of actively trying to promote work enjoyment among staff members. The view is that as long as staff do a good job, then agency services will be provided appropriately whether staff members enjoy their work or not. A premise of this training session is that such a view is counterproductive to effective supervision, especially when considering the quality of agency services over the long run.

SHOW SLIDE 8.2

Slide 8.2: Importance of Promoting Staff Work Enjoyment

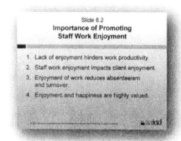

IMPORTANCE OF WORK ENJOYMENT

One reason staff work enjoyment is important is that a significant lack of enjoyment, or workplace discontent, hinders work productivity. When staff members are displeased about things that regularly occur on the job, much of their time and energy is directed to those things. Staff members spend time trying to find ways to resolve the sources of their discontent or frequently spend time complaining about their jobs. Time spent in these activities detracts from time that should be spent getting the job done.

? QUESTION TRAINEES

Ask trainees if they have ever been in a situation in which certain staff seem to constantly complain about various aspects of the job. Then prompt brief discussion about how the complaining can interfere with staff working diligently to perform their job duties.

Another reason staff members' work enjoyment is important is that their enjoyment tends to foster enjoyment among agency clients. Staff members who appear happy and upbeat make for a much more enjoyable social climate for clients than those who act disgruntled and frequently complain. Staff enjoyment similarly affects a supervisor's quality of work life.

? QUESTION TRAINEES

Ask trainees whether they prefer working more with staff members who appear to enjoy their jobs and seem content or with those who appear not to enjoy their jobs and are frequently complaining to the supervisor or other staff members. Prompt brief discussion around the issue that most of us prefer to work with people who are upbeat and positive in their actions.

Still another reason for trying to help staff members enjoy their work pertains to a problem many of us have dealt with: *staff absenteeism and turnover*. Though many factors relate to absenteeism and turnover, one of the most significant is staff members' lack of enjoyment of their jobs. In short, the more staff members enjoy their jobs, the more they will show up for work and the longer they will stay.

The final reason for emphasizing staff work enjoyment is value based. We simply value people enjoying their work and generally being content on the job. Most of us, as well as our staff, spend a large portion of our adult lives at work. Our lives are enriched overall if we enjoy our work life as much as reasonably possible.

? QUESTION TRAINEES

Ask trainees if they get up in the morning and look forward to going to work. Note that most people respond to this question by saying "sometimes." That is, *sometimes* they get up in the morning and look forward to going to work.

SHOW SLIDE 8.3 ▶

Slide 8.3: Goal for Staff Work Enjoyment

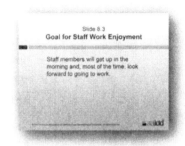

Our goal for promoting staff members' enjoyment of their work is that most of the time they will get up in the morning and look forward to going to work. In an ideal world, staff members would always look forward to their jobs. However, due to the nature of *work*, it is likely that there will always be some things that people dislike about a job. That is why we realistically aim for the goal of staff members getting up and looking forward to going to work at least more often than not.

Specific Strategies for Promoting Staff Work Enjoyment

THINGS SUPERVISORS CANNOT DO

There are, of course, some job aspects affecting staff work enjoyment that a supervisor has no control over. Often supervisors have little, if any, control over the amount of pay staff members receive or when they receive raises. How much one is paid for a job can certainly affect work enjoyment.

Sometimes the work schedule affects work enjoyment, such as for staff members who do not like to work on weekends or holidays. Many supervisors, such as those working in residential settings, must schedule staff members to work weekends and holidays even when they know certain staff members really do not like it.

FOCUS ON WHAT CAN BE DONE

However, there are also many things supervisors *can do* that affect work enjoyment. We will focus on those things and simply accept that there are some other things that supervisors cannot control. Keep in mind, though, that supervisory actions to promote staff work enjoyment should occur in conjunction with actions to improve and support quality work performance. Promoting work enjoyment but not achieving quality work would not represent effective supervision.

SHOW SLIDE 8.4 ▶

Slide 8.4: What Supervisors Can Do to Promote Staff Work Enjoyment

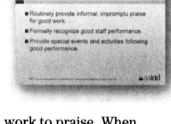

WAYS TO PROMOTE WORK ENJOYMENT

One thing supervisors can do to promote staff enjoyment on the job is to make it standard practice to commend or praise staff members for their good work. We are referring here primarily to what is considered *impromptu praise*. Whenever supervisors happen to observe commendable work performance, praise for the work can occur in an impromptu or on-the-spot manner.

Supervisors should constantly be looking for good work to praise. When staff members receive praise from their supervisor about their work, they usually feel good about their work and themselves. Feeling good on the job represents one source of enjoyment.

Impromptu praise represents a form of informal feedback. As a type of feedback, it should only be presented when it is sincere, as we discussed before. This is also a type of feedback that does not require all the steps of diagnostic feedback that we discussed earlier. It merely requires that a supervisor let a staff member know specifically what he or she did well on the job.

Because a supervisor's job is usually very busy, some supervisors make special arrangements to ensure they spend some time every day, or at least every few days, praising staff for some part of their work performance. For example, some supervisors list "praise good work performance of at least one staff member" on their daily to-do list along with other important supervisory tasks.

TRAINEE ACTIVITY

Distribute Activity Sheet 8.1 to each trainee. Read the instructions at the top of the sheet. Instruct trainees that they should work in small groups and discuss how to complete the activity sheet. However, note that each trainee should develop his or her system for encouraging supervisor praise by completing the sheet. After sufficient time for each trainee to complete the sheet, instruct trainees to share what they developed with each other in their groups. Subsequently (after a maximum of 15 minutes to complete the entire task) ask several trainees to share what they heard from another trainee that they thought was a good way to encourage supervisor praise of staff work (i.e., the trainees should share what they heard from another trainee, not what the trainees have developed themselves). Thank the trainees for sharing, though making sure the systems that are shared fulfill the intent of the task (i.e., it specifically identifies a work performance to monitor and praise, the frequency with which praise will be provided, and the plan for documenting that the praise was provided).

PRAISE WORK PERFORMANCE TO OTHERS

Those of you who shared ways to commend a staff member's performance that you heard from another trainee just illustrated a way to praise performance that is more indirect than what we have been discussing but nonetheless important. That is, you indirectly praised your colleague's performance by commending the person's actions to others instead of providing the praise directly to the staff member. By indicating to the rest of us that you liked what the respective trainee did, you in essence commended that person's performance.

Praising staff work performance can also occur in other ways besides telling the staff members about their good work or telling others about their good work in an impromptu or informal manner. For example, upon noticing some particularly praiseworthy performance, supervisors can later send brief notes, memos, or e-mail messages to staff members for the sole purpose of commending their performance.

Because these ways to commend staff performance are somewhat informal, they can be done at essentially any time. Providing impromptu praise whenever a supervisor happens to see a staff member do something well on the job is applicable to almost any job situation.

Slide 8.4: What Supervisors Can Do to Promote Staff Work Enjoyment

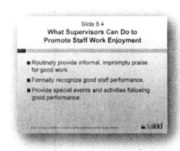

There are also more formal ways to praise good staff performance. One way pertains to something that most of you are familiar with in your agency. Most agencies have some type of formal recognition procedures: an "Employee of the Month," an "Annual Outstanding Staff Award," or a "Good Attendance Certificate." Formal recognition procedures are a nice way to commend staff performance and can help staff members feel good about their work.

However, there are also special considerations when using formal recognition procedures if they are to fulfill the intended purpose of helping staff members feel good about their work and promoting work enjoyment.

Slide 8.5: Special Considerations for Formal Recognition Procedures

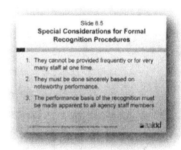

One consideration with formal recognition procedures is that they usually cannot be presented to the staff very frequently, or they can only be presented to a small number of staff at a given time. For example, presenting an "Employee of the Year Award" obviously is not going to occur very often or for very many staff members. Hence, these procedures should be used *in addition to* the more informal ways to commend staff performance that should be in place routinely.

Additionally, formal recognition should be done sincerely, and the recognition should be clearly based on commendable performance that has been directly observed. Providing recognition based on something other than commendable performance can seriously hinder job enjoyment among many staff.

To illustrate further, in some cases formal recognition has been provided to a staff member because a supervisor has a familial or other special relationship with the staff member, even though the staff member's performance has been less than adequate. When staff members become aware that a co-worker's work is being formally commended when they know the individual's performance is often inadequate, their reaction is not very favorable.

Staff members also tend to lose respect for a supervisor who is responsible for such action. For this reason, it is always important to specify the good work behavior of the staff member receiving the recognition such that all agency staff members are aware that the award is given for good performance and nothing else.

SHOW SLIDE 8.4 AGAIN

Slide 8.4: What Supervisors Can Do to Promote Staff Work Enjoyment

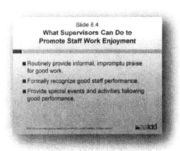

Another more formal way to promote workplace enjoyment is through special events that the staff members enjoy. Again, many of you are familiar with these. They may involve a special dinner for staff, a lottery drawing in which selected staff members win gift certificates, or a fun recreational activity for staff.

As with other ways to commend staff and effectively promote work enjoyment, special events must be conducted in certain ways. Specifically, they must be held in response to some nice things that an agency's staff have done on the job, and the reason for the event must be made apparent to all staff members. This way, the event helps not only with staff work enjoyment but also to support desired work performance.

CONDUCT COMPETENCY CHECK

Conduct the competency check using Competency Check Form 8.1.

Slide 8.1
Evidence-Based Supervisory Strategies

1. Specify staff performance expectations.
2. Monitor staff performance.
3. Provide feedback based on performance.
4. Provide performance-based and competency-based training as needed.

Slide 8.2
Importance of Promoting Staff Work Enjoyment

1. Lack of enjoyment hinders work productivity.
2. Staff work enjoyment impacts client enjoyment.
3. Enjoyment of work reduces absenteeism and turnover.
4. Enjoyment and happiness are highly valued.

Slide 8.3
Goal for Staff Work Enjoyment

Staff members will get up in the morning and, most of the time, look forward to going to work.

Slide 8.4
What Supervisors Can Do to Promote Staff Work Enjoyment

- Routinely provide informal, impromptu praise for good work.
- Formally recognize good staff performance.
- Provide special events and activities following good performance.

Slide 8.5
Special Considerations for Formal Recognition Procedures

1. They cannot be provided frequently or for very many staff at one time.

2. They must be done sincerely based on noteworthy performance.

3. The performance basis of the recognition must be made apparent to all agency staff members.

MODULE 8 ACTIVITY SHEET 8.1

Promoting Quality Work Performance With Enjoyment

Trainee name: _____ Date: _____

INSTRUCTIONS

Develop a system for a supervisor to praise an aspect of good work of staff on at least a weekly basis. Answer the following questions in a way sufficiently specific such that it could be given to a new supervisor so that he or she would know what to do. First, describe some aspect of staff work duties that should be performed routinely (e.g., interacting positively with clients). Second, describe how often at a minimum the supervisor should praise at least one staff member for the performance area designated in question 1. Third, describe how a supervisor could keep track of fulfilling the responsibility of praising the performance within the specified schedule (e.g., setting up a chart for recording the presentation of praise according to the schedule).

1. Which staff work duties will be monitored in order to allow for commendation or praise to be provided routinely?

2. What is the minimum frequency for praising the performance?

3. How will it be documented that the supervisor provided praise at the designated frequency?

MODULE 8 COMPETENCY CHECK

Promoting Quality Work Performance With Enjoyment

TRAINER INSTRUCTIONS

- Distribute Competency Check Form 8.1 to each trainee.
- Instruct the trainees to gather in small groups at their tables.
- Read the instructions at the top of the form.
- Instruct trainees to follow the instructions on the form and jointly complete Competency Check Form 8.1.
- Inform trainees that a completed copy of Competency Check Form 8.1 should be turned in for each group of trainees.
- Allow no more than 15 minutes for the activity.

MASTERY CRITERION

Each group of trainees must answer each question on Competency Check Form 8.1.

MODULE COMPETENCY CHECK FORM 8.1:
PROMOTING QUALITY WORK PERFORMANCE WITH ENJOYMENT

Encouraging Formal Recognition

Trainees' names (all trainees in the group): _____ Date: _____

INSTRUCTIONS

Develop a system for providing formal recognition of a staff member's good work on a monthly or quarterly basis. Answer the following questions in a way sufficiently specific such that it could be given to a new supervisor so that he or she would know what to do. First, describe some aspect of staff work duties that should be performed routinely. Second, describe in detail how formal recognition could be given to at least a staff member for the performance designated in question 1.

1. Which staff work duties will be monitored in order to allow for formal recognition to be given monthly or quarterly?

2. What is the procedure for giving formal recognition? Describe this in detail.

MODULE 9

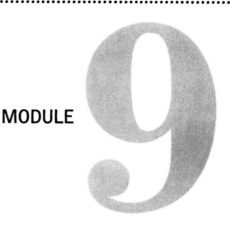

Reducing Workplace Discontent

The following will be covered on day 2 of training.

Objectives

Upon completion of this module, trainees should be able to do the following:

1. Describe four supervisory activities that often cause staff discontent.
2. Describe four supervisory activities that often prevent staff discontent.
3. Describe a four-step process for making work tasks that are highly disliked by staff more enjoyable to perform.

Method

1. Presentation on overall concept of reducing discontent: *3 minutes*
2. Presentation and trainee discussion on supervisory activities that tend to cause discontent among staff: *10 minutes*
3. Presentation and trainee discussion on supervisory activities for preventing discontent among staff: *10 minutes*
4. Presentation and trainee discussion on reducing discontent with performing certain job duties: *12 minutes*
5. Competency check and follow-up discussion: *25 minutes*

Competency Check, Materials, and Total Training Time

1. Competency check: Completion of Competency Check Form 9.1
2. Materials
   a. PowerPoint presentation equipment (LCD, computer, curriculum CD) or
   b. Overhead projector and copies of Slides 9.1, 9.2, 9.3, 9.4, and 9.5
   c. Competency Check Form 9.1
3. Total training time: *1 hour*

Reducing Workplace Discontent

Essentially every job has good things and bad things associated with it. The more good things there are with a job relative to the bad things, generally the more staff members enjoy the job.

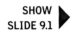

SHOW SLIDE 9.1

INCREASE GOOD THINGS AND DECREASE BAD THINGS

Slide 9.1: Maximizing Work Enjoyment: Increasing the Positives and Decreasing the Negatives

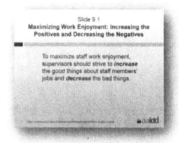

To maximize work enjoyment among the staff, supervisors should strive to increase the good things about a job and decrease the bad things. To this point, we have been primarily discussing ways supervisors can increase the good things about staff's job. Most importantly, we have stressed supervisors should *routinely* praise quality staff performance. We have also noted the importance of periodically providing special recognition for a job well done.

Supervisors can also affect staff work enjoyment by decreasing bad things associated with a job. When supervisors successfully decrease negative aspects of a job for the staff, then their overall enjoyment of the job increases. This session focuses on how supervisors can decrease some of the things staff members often dislike about their jobs. The intent is to reduce common sources of staff discontent with human service jobs.

IMPORTANCE OF HOW SUPERVISORS INTERACT WITH STAFF

Reducing Staff Discontent With Supervisory Actions

One source of staff discontent in the workplace that supervisors can have direct control over is how they interact with staff. How supervisors interact with staff can either cause or prevent discontent among staff.

QUESTION TRAINEES

Ask trainees if they have ever worked for a supervisor who caused them discontent because of the way the supervisor interacted with, or treated, them. Then ask for some examples of what the supervisor did that they disliked. Be careful to maintain professionalism during the discussion (e.g., make sure trainees refrain from specifically identifying any supervisors with whom the trainees had difficulty). Use the examples to illustrate how a supervisor's interaction with them impacted their work enjoyment at times, and the same types of situations can exist with any supervisor's interactions with staff.

Surveys of support staff in human service agencies have shown that there are several ways supervisors interact with staff that frequently result in staff discontent.

SHOW SLIDE 9.2

Slide 9.2: Supervisor Activities Frequently Resulting in Staff Discontent

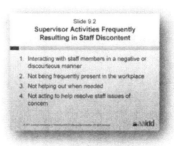

While discussing the slide in the following section, relate the points to any examples mentioned by the trainees that are the same or similar to the points in the slide.

SUPERVISORY ACTIVITIES CAUSING STAFF DISCONTENT

The most common supervisory activity that causes job discontent is a supervisor *frequently interacting with staff in a negative manner*. This is exemplified by frequently criticizing what staff members do or criticizing the staff members themselves. It is also illustrated by a supervisor's lack of basic social courtesy, such as not speaking to a staff member when passing in a hallway or not responding to his or her question or comment.

A second supervisory activity that results in staff discontent is *infrequent presence*—that is, the staff members rarely see their supervisor in their workplace. Previously the importance of supervisor visibility or presence in the workplace was noted. One reason for stressing supervisor presence is that when the supervisor is *not* around very much, it often becomes disconcerting for the staff.

A third and related supervisory activity that staff members frequently dislike is *failure to help out* when needed. Supervisors who never, or rarely, help staff members fulfill their duties, particularly during very busy or otherwise difficult times, are usually not viewed very favorably by the staff. The unfavorable impact on the staff can cause serious discontent.

A fourth supervisory activity resulting in staff discontent is *failure to act*—that is, when a staff member approaches the supervisor with a job need, the supervisor does nothing to address the need. The supervisor may say the situation will be looked into but rarely does anything to try to resolve the issue of concern.

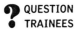 **QUESTION TRAINEES**

Ask trainees if they have ever worked for a supervisor who rarely, if ever, attempted to resolve a problem for which they had asked the supervisor for help. Also ask if they have ever worked for a supervisor who often said he or she would take care of a problem situation but never did anything. Then note that in those situations, the trainees probably did not have a very favorable view of the supervisor.

MODULE 9: REDUCING WORKPLACE DISCONTENT | 99

SHOW SLIDE 9.3

SUPERVISORY ACTIVITIES PREVENTING DISCONTENT

Slide 9.3: Supervisor Activities for Preventing Staff Discontent

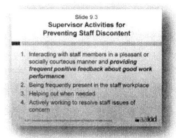

To prevent or reduce staff discontent in the workplace, supervisors should strive to act in certain ways during the daily job routine. The ways noted on the slide represent supervisor activities that many staff members have reported helped them to enjoy working for a supervisor. As you can see, these ways are in direct contrast to the supervisor activities just described that often represent sources of discontent.

The most commonly reported supervisor activity that enhances day-to-day job enjoyment is the supervisor interacting with the staff in a pleasant or socially courteous manner. Socially courteous behavior involves many things, and we cannot cover all of them here. However, we do stress the basics of social courtesy by supervisors, such as greeting a staff member when passing in a hallway, responding when a staff member initiates an interaction, and attempting to answer questions that a staff member poses.

QUESTION TRAINEES

Ask trainees to give some examples of how supervisors can interact with staff members that represent pleasant or socially courteous behavior. Make sure to relate what the trainees report to the following discussion (e.g., when discussing the ways to interact, note if a respective way was already identified by one or more trainees).

IMPORTANCE OF FEEDBACK

One of the most straightforward ways for supervisors to interact with a staff member in a pleasant manner is to *give positive feedback* about good aspects of his or her work as emphasized previously. Positive feedback is almost always favorably received by a staff member, especially if it is presented sincerely and specifically related to a staff member's work activity, which was also discussed earlier.

In emphasizing frequent presentation of positive feedback, it should be remembered that staff members must be held accountable for their work behavior. We note this because we do not want to leave the impression that supervisors should provide *only* positive feedback.

When a staff member performs some aspect of work in an unacceptable manner, corrective feedback must be provided to improve the performance. However, to minimize staff discontent, supervisors should provide much more positive than negative feedback to the staff.

Using the diagnostic feedback protocol we practiced previously helps ensure that whenever corrective feedback is provided, positive feedback is also presented for aspects of work that is performed well.

BE PRESENT

A second means of preventing staff discontent is for a supervisor to make sure he or she is *frequently present* in the staff work area. This is especially true for supervisors who work in a location separate from the staff.

HELP OUT

Being frequently present in the staff work area has the additional benefit of giving the supervisor opportunities to periodically help staff members perform some of their duties. *Helping out* represents another way to reduce staff discontent. Of course, supervisors must be careful about how much time they spend helping staff members perform their duties. Supervisors have their own jobs to do and should not help with staff duties so much that they neglect their own jobs. A good rule of thumb is that on average, supervisors should help staff with aspects of their job at least some every week.

ACT ON STAFF CONCERNS

A fourth way to reduce staff discontent is for a supervisor to make sure to *act* in response to a staff member's expression of a need for assistance. Supervisors should strive to resolve problematic situations for the staff by taking whatever action is appropriate and possible. When a supervisor has no control over a situation causing concern for a staff member, the supervisor should at least acknowledge the concern and that the particular issue is one the supervisor is not likely to be able to remedy.

Reducing Staff Discontent With Features Inherent in Certain Job Duties

A major source of staff discontent in the workplace beyond how a supervisor interacts with the staff pertains more directly to the specific jobs of support staff. As with most jobs, there are often some duties expected of support staff in the human services that simply are not very enjoyable to perform.

QUESTION TRAINEES

Ask trainees to name some job duties that they have found that the staff members (or themselves when working in a support role) often dislike having to perform.

A good way to reduce staff discontent is to alter job duties that are disliked to make them more enjoyable to perform or, at least, less disliked.

REFER TO TRAINEE EXAMPLES

Summarize some of the examples just provided by the trainees. Note that if those specific job duties could be made more enjoyable for staff to perform, then some sources of discontent for staff could be reduced or removed from the workplace.

Realistically, supervisors will not have the time or be able to make all staff duties very enjoyable to perform. However, supervisors can strive to make certain, highly disliked duties more enjoyable for the staff to fulfill.

SHOW SLIDE 9.4

Slide 9.4: How to Make Highly Disliked Work Tasks More Enjoyable for Staff

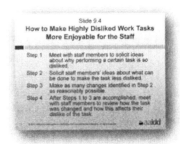

STEP 1

When a supervisor becomes aware that a certain job duty is highly disliked by the staff, several steps can be taken to make the duty nicer for the staff to perform. Step 1 is to meet with staff members and prompt them for ideas about what *specifically* makes them dislike the job duty.

STEP 2

Step 2 is to solicit opinions from the staff about how the disliked aspects of the task could reasonably be altered to make it less disliked. Supervisors usually will also have to come up with their own ideas of how to change the job duty to make it less disliked or solicit ideas from other supervisors or executive personnel.

STEPS 3 AND 4

Step 3 is to make as many of the changes as possible to make the task more pleasant. Step 4 is to subsequently meet with staff members again to review what was done and how it has impacted their discontent with the particular duty.

Before illustrating how these steps can work with an actual job duty that staff members reported they disliked, the importance of Step 4 warrants elaboration. Sometimes the actions taken by a supervisor will be only partially effective in making a job duty more enjoyable to perform, or maybe they will not be very effective at all. However, by reviewing the actions taken with the staff, two beneficial outcomes are likely to occur.

First, more ideas of what can be done to make the duty more desirable may be identified. Second, even if the actions taken were not very successful, the staff members often become appreciative of the supervisor making the effort to listen to them and trying to make things better. Being appreciative of a supervisor's efforts represents a good thing within the staff's overall work life and, therefore, is something worth promoting.

Review the steps on the overhead.

SHOW SLIDE 9.5

Slide 9.5: Example of Making a Disliked Job Task More Liked

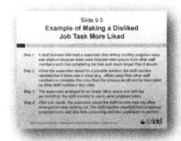

SUMMARIZE EXAMPLE

With the example just noted, the staff member initially reported to her supervisor that completing client-progress notes each month was the most disliked task of all her job duties. After all the steps were followed, the staff member then reported that completing progress notes was no longer the most disliked of all her duties and was even more liked than a number of other duties.

The case illustrated is only one example of how the steps can be taken in an attempt to make a highly disliked work task more enjoyable for a staff member to perform. Of course, what is most disliked by respective staff members will vary, as will what is done to make the task less disliked. The point here is supervisors can take specific steps in a systematic manner to reduce some workplace discontent that is associated with performing a certain job duty.

CONDUCT COMPETENCY CHECK

Conduct the competency check using Competency Check Form 9.1. After trainees complete the competency check, have each group of trainees summarize their answers to the questions on the form for the rest of the class. If necessary, redirect trainee presentations to make sure that their answers specifically address each respective question.

Slide 9.1
Maximizing Work Enjoyment: Increasing the Positives and Decreasing the Negatives

To maximize staff work enjoyment, supervisors should strive to *increase* the good things about staff members' jobs and *decrease* the bad things.

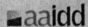

Slide 9.2
Supervisor Activities Frequently Resulting in Staff Discontent

1. Interacting with staff members in a negative or discourteous manner
2. Not being frequently present in the workplace
3. Not helping out when needed
4. Not acting to help resolve staff issues of concern

Slide 9.3
Supervisor Activities for Preventing Staff Discontent

1. Interacting with staff members in a pleasant or socially courteous manner and *providing frequent positive feedback about good work performance*
2. Being frequently present in the staff workplace
3. Helping out when needed
4. Actively working to resolve staff issues of concern

Slide 9.4
How to Make Highly Disliked Work Tasks More Enjoyable for the Staff

Step 1   Meet with staff members to solicit ideas about why performing a certain task is so disliked.

Step 2   Solicit staff members' ideas about what can be done to make the task less disliked.

Step 3   Make as many changes identified in Step 2 as reasonably possible.

Step 4   After Steps 1 to 3 are accomplished, meet with staff members to review how the task was changed and how this affects their dislike of the task.

Slide 9.5
Example of Making a Disliked Job Task More Liked

Step 1 A staff member informed a supervisor that writing monthly progress notes was disliked because there were frequent interruptions from other staff members such that completing the task took much longer than it should.

Step 2 When the supervisor asked for a possible solution, the staff member reported that if there was a place (e.g., office) away from other staff members to complete the notes then the process would not be interrupted by other staff members very often.

Step 3 The supervisor arranged for an empty office space one half-day per month for the staff member to use to write progress notes.

Step 4 After one month, the supervisor asked the staff member how the office arrangement was working out. The staff member reported that completing progress notes was less time consuming and less unpleasant to perform.

© 2011 American Association on Intellectual and Developmental Disabilities. All rights reserved.

MODULE 9 COMPETENCY CHECK
Reducing Workplace Discontent

TRAINER INSTRUCTIONS

- Distribute Competency Check Form 9.1 to each trainee.
- Instruct the trainees to gather in small groups at their tables.
- Read the instructions at the top of the form.
- Instruct trainees to follow the instructions on the form and jointly complete Competency Check Form 9.1.
- Inform trainees that each of their groups will be asked to summarize their answers in class.
- Inform trainees that a completed copy of Competency Check Form 9.1 should be turned in for each group of trainees.
- Allow no more than 25 minutes for the activity.

MASTERY CRITERION

Each group of trainees must answer each question on Competency Check Form 9.1.

MODULE 9 COMPETENCY CHECK FORM 9.1

Reducing Workplace Discontent

Trainees' names (all trainees in the group): _____ Date: _____

INSTRUCTIONS

Describe how to make a work task that is very disliked by staff members more enjoyable for them to perform. Answer each question below.

1. In your experience, which work task is highly disliked by one or more staff members?

2. What specific aspects of the task make it unpleasant? Provide your ideas (or those of staff if known).

3. How can the aspects identified in question 2 be altered to make the task more enjoyable to perform?

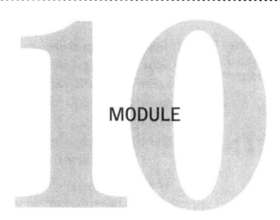

MODULE 10

Resolving Recurrent Performance Problems

The following will be covered on day 2 of training.

Objectives

Upon completion of this module, trainees should be able to do the following:

1. Describe four primary reasons for recurrent performance problems among staff.
2. Describe the primary supervisory action for resolving each of the four main reasons for recurrent performance problems.
3. Describe five guidelines for using disciplinary action effectively.

Method

1. Presentation on review of evidence-based supervision: *5 minutes*
2. Presentation and trainee discussion on four primary reasons for recurrent performance problems among staff: *20 minutes*
3. Presentation and trainee discussion on using disciplinary action to resolve recurrent performance problems: *25 minutes*
4. Competency check: *10 minutes*

Competency Check, Materials, and Total Training Time

1. Competency check: Completion of Competency Check Form 10.1
2. Materials
   a. PowerPoint presentation equipment (LCD, computer, curriculum CD) or
   b. Overhead projector and copies of Slides 10.1, 10.2, 10.3, 10.4, 10.5, 10.6, 10.7, and 10.8
   c. Competency Check Form 10.1
3. Total training time: *1 hour*

Resolving Recurrent Performance Problems

REVIEW EVIDENCE-BASED SUPERVISION

If the evidence-based supervisory procedures discussed to this point are consistently practiced by supervisors, support staff will usually perform their duties with quality. Support staff will also likely experience a rather enjoyable quality of work life.

SHOW SLIDE 10.1

Slide 10.1: Summary of Evidence-Based Supervisory Strategies

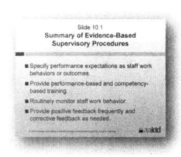

To briefly review one more time, supervisors should make sure performance expectations of staff members are clearly specified, staff members are well trained to perform their duties, staff work activities are routinely monitored, and positive feedback is provided frequently along with corrective feedback as necessary.

SHOW SLIDE 10.2

Slide 10.2: Making Work Life Enjoyable and Reducing Discontent

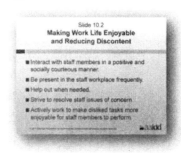

Supervisors should also take specific actions to promote enjoyment and prevent potential discontent in the workplace. Such actions include interacting with staff in a socially courteous manner, frequently being present in the staff work area, helping out when needed, striving to resolve staff concerns, and actively working to make disliked tasks more enjoyable for staff.

PURPOSE OF SESSION

Although this approach to supervision is the most readily available means through which supervisors can promote a high-quality, enjoyable work environment, it is not perfect. There will be times, despite a supervisor's proficient and diligent efforts, when some staff members will have recurrent problems performing certain job duties. This session focuses on how supervisors can deal with persistent staff performance problems.

SHOW SLIDE 10.3

Slide 10.3: First Step for Resolving Recurring Performance Problems

FIRST STEP: CORRECTIVE FEEDBACK

When a staff member is repeatedly demonstrating problematic performance, the first supervisory action is to provide *corrective feedback*. As discussed previously, corrective feedback informs the staff member that what he or she is doing is not acceptable and specifies how his or her performance should be corrected. It is also most beneficial if the corrective feedback is supplemented with positive feedback about related work behavior that is being completed adequately.

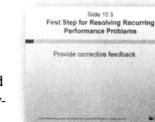

If improvement does not result after corrective feedback has been presented on two or three occasions, then a supervisor must take additional steps to improve the performance. What a supervisor specifically does should be based on the supervisor's assessment regarding *why* the staff member's work is inadequate.

QUESTION TRAINEES

Ask trainees to think about a staff member who persistently did not perform a certain work duty adequately. What do they think is the reason for that person's lack of acceptable work behavior? Ask several trainees to share their thoughts with the entire class. When presenting the following information, relate the discussed reasons for problematic performance to what the trainees noted (i.e., the reasons offered by the trainees probably fall within one of the following areas).

SHOW SLIDE 10.4

Slide 10.4: Key Reasons for Recurring Performance Problems and Required Supervisor Action

PROVIDE TRAINING

Inadequate staff work behavior usually occurs for one of several key reasons. One reason is that staff members do not know *how* to do the task. Either these staff members did not receive necessary training or the training was not carried out effectively. In such cases, the required supervisory action is to adequately train the staff. The training should be performance based and competency based, as we have practiced in Module 7.

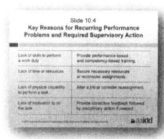

CONSIDER LACK OF RESOURCES

A second reason for inadequate staff work behavior is that the staff member does not have time to do a task due to other assigned duties or does not have the resources to do the task. Lack of resources usually means a staff member does not have ready access to necessary materials to do the duty. For example, a staff member in a group home may have minimal leisure materials available, making it difficult to promote evening leisure engagement among clients because there is little for the clients to do.

QUESTION TRAINEES

Ask trainees to give some examples of where they have seen inadequate staff performance due to a lack of time or resources for staff to do the job.

REVIEW RESOURCES

The required supervisory action when insufficient time or resources appear to be the cause of problematic staff performance is to secure the necessary resources. If the supervisor does not have the capability of securing the resources, such as not being able to obtain more staff or reduce other competing duties of staff, then the assigned duties of staff must be reconsidered. A staff member should not be put in the position of being expected to do a job task when there are not sufficient resources.

It should also be noted that caution is needed when attributing a performance problem to lack of time or resources. This is particularly the case when a given staff member says that he or she cannot do the job adequately because there is not enough time. Sometimes this is a valid reason and sometimes it is simply an excuse to avoid performing the duty. Supervisors need to be sufficiently familiar with and knowledgeable about the work situation to determine if lack of resources is a true problem or not.

INDIVIDUAL STAFF ISSUES

A third reason for a recurring performance problem may arise from issues that are idiosyncratic to a particular staff member. For example, sometimes a staff person's health or physical challenges prohibit him or her from performing a certain duty proficiently.

? QUESTION TRAINEES

Ask trainees if they have experienced situations in which a staff member could not physically perform an assigned job duty. Ask several trainees to share the experience. Make sure to maintain professional confidentiality by not identifying any staff person by name.

INDIVIDUALIZE SUPERVISORY ACTION

Because of the individualized nature of this reason for a recurring performance problem, the required supervisory action will also have to be individualized. The action will likely require upper management assistance to determine if, for example, the staff member can be relieved of a certain duty or the duty can be altered to make it easier to do. In the most extreme situation, a decision may have to be made as to whether the staff member should remain employed in the agency when he or she cannot physically do parts of the job.

Although resolving a recurring performance problem due to physical challenges of a staff member may require different solutions, one thing is certain: Job expectations should not be allowed to continue unchanged when it is clear that a staff member physically cannot fulfill the expectations. This is not fair to the staff person or to the clients who are recipients of the agency's services.

LACK OF STAFF MOTIVATION

The fourth reason for a recurring performance problem is probably the most common and most difficult for a supervisor: The staff member knows how to do the job task and can do the task but lacks motivation to do it or do it right. In these cases, supervisors need to take more severe, corrective action.

Severe Corrective Procedures: Disciplinary Action

Severe corrective procedures involve what is usually referred to as *disciplinary action*. Essentially every human service agency has a policy that dictates how disciplinary action should be used for various performance problems.

QUESTION TRAINEES

Ask several trainees to briefly describe how disciplinary action policies are designed in their agency.

SHOW SLIDE 10.5

GOAL OF DISCIPLINARY ACTION

TWO WAYS TO APPLY DISCIPLINARY ACTION

Slide 10.5: Goal of Disciplinary Action

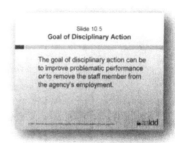

From a basic supervisory perspective, the goal of disciplinary action is two-fold: to improve problematic performance or, if improvement does not result, remove the staff member from the agency's employment.

Typically, disciplinary action should be applied in one of two ways. One way pertains to work behavior that is identified by an agency as totally unacceptable, such as abusing a client, being intoxicated at work, or stealing client property. When this behavior is known to occur, then the resulting disciplinary action usually should be to remove the employee through job termination.

The second way pertains to problems with work behavior that are less serious but occur repeatedly. In these cases, disciplinary action usually involves beginning with a somewhat mild but formal corrective action such as a documented, formal counseling session with the staff member. If the problems recur, then more severe action is taken, such as a formal written warning. More severe action continues to be taken if the problems continue, ultimately resulting in termination of the staff member's employment.

The concern here is with those performance problems that are not so severe that they warrant immediate job termination but nonetheless need correction.

SHOW SLIDE 10.6

FIRST GUIDELINE FOR DISCIPLINARY ACTION

Slide 10.6: Effective Use of Disciplinary Action

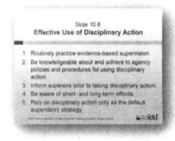

There are five guidelines for effectively using disciplinary action to correct problematic work behavior that has not responded to corrective feedback. The first is that disciplinary action works best if evidence-based supervision is practiced by a supervisor. All the things we have talked about for promoting quality work performance and enjoyment should be routinely practiced. If they are, then disciplinary action will not be needed very often and when it is needed, it will be more effective.

If sound, evidence-based supervision is not routinely practiced and disciplinary action is regularly used in attempts to improve staff performance, then a supervisor will likely encounter serious difficulties.

SHOW SLIDE 10.7

Slide 10.7: Problems With Frequently Relying on Disciplinary Action

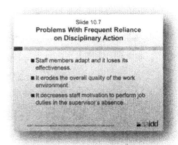

QUESTION TRAINEES

Ask trainees if they have seen some problems when disciplinary action has been used frequently in an agency. Ask several trainees to share their experiences with the rest of the class. Then relate their experiences to the points on Slide 10.7 during the following discussion.

PROBLEMS WITH TOO MUCH DISCIPLINARY ACTION

One difficulty with frequent reliance on disciplinary action is that the more disciplinary action is used, the more staff members get used to it. Hence, disciplinary action loses its effectiveness for improving work behavior. In contrast, if staff members are used to a supervisor giving frequent positive feedback and corrective feedback only as needed, then when disciplinary action is used on occasion it usually evokes serious staff attention and response.

A second problem with frequent reliance on disciplinary action is that by its nature disciplinary action is punitive for staff. Its negative features represent a bad thing in the staff's work environment such that if used too often then it seriously erodes the quality of the work environment. In short, frequent use of disciplinary action detracts from efforts to motivate staff members to work diligently and to enjoy their work.

A third difficulty with overreliance on disciplinary action is that it tends to create an environment in which staff members are motivated to do certain parts of their job *only to avoid the action by the supervisor.* A staff member will perform acceptably when the supervisor is around to avoid the supervisor catching him or her performing inadequately and taking disciplinary action. However, when the supervisor is not around, there is no motivation for the staff person to perform acceptably and his or her performance will be less than adequate.

SHOW SLIDE 10.6 AGAIN

Slide 10.6: Effective Use of Disciplinary Action

Again, the first guideline for effective use of disciplinary action is the point we have been making: It should be used in conjunction with routine application of evidence-based supervisory practices. Evidence-based supervisory actions should be the norm and disciplinary action should be only a periodic supplement to how a supervisor works with staff.

SECOND GUIDELINE FOR DISCIPLINARY ACTION

The second guideline is that supervisors must become very knowledgeable about an agency's policies and procedures for how to use disciplinary action and must carefully follow those policies and procedures. Following agency policies and procedures helps make sure disciplinary action is applied consistently and fairly. Following appropriate rules when using disciplinary action also makes it work more effectively.

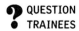
QUESTION TRAINEES

Ask trainees if they are aware of any situations in which disciplinary action taken with a staff member was subsequently overturned or withdrawn by management or personnel officers. Then ask several trainees to share any negative implications for the workplace when a disciplinary action was later negated. Prompt trainees to discuss how this situation is rarely good for the work environment (use the following guidelines).

A common reason that disciplinary action is overturned is that the supervisor taking the action did not follow agency policies or procedures. Every time a disciplinary action is overturned or withdrawn, it detracts from the future effectiveness of such action. The staff begins to realize that any negative sanctions inherent in disciplinary action will not actually occur. Additionally, the supervisor's credibility with the staff can be eroded and the supervisor's future actions are less likely to impact staff performance.

THIRD GUIDELINE FOR DISCIPLINARY ACTION

The third guideline for use of disciplinary action is for the supervisor to inform his or her superiors *prior to* taking the action with a staff member. In this manner, the superiors will be aware of the reason for the action and can be in a better situation to support the supervisor's action. In contrast, if the superiors first hear about the action from the staff member who is disgruntled about the action, then the superiors are less able to support the supervisor because they are unaware of the supervisor's reasons. The latter situation makes it more likely that the action will be overturned.

FOURTH GUIDELINE FOR DISCIPLINARY ACTION

The fourth guideline is more of something that the supervisor should be aware of than something that needs to be done. Specifically, supervisors should be aware that disciplinary action—and especially actions that are severe, such as job suspension or termination—have both short- and long-term effects.

TWO EFFECTS OF DISCIPLINARY ACTION

The short-term effect is that often supervisors may be viewed in a negative light by the staff member's peers. Other workers may feel sorry for the staff person receiving disciplinary action and question the need for the supervisor's negative actions. However, this is a usually short-lived effect, especially if the supervisor routinely practices evidence-based supervision and adheres to appropriate policies regarding use of disciplinary action.

The long-term effect of appropriate use of disciplinary action is that it can improve problematic performance. Additionally, the staff will typically respect a supervisor who actively works to improve inadequate performance of his or her respective staff. Most staff members are usually aware when one of their peers is performing inadequately and that it is a supervisor's job to correct that performance. Most staff members also prefer working for a supervisor who will take action to correct unacceptable performance rather than a supervisor who takes no formal action.

MODULE 10: RESOLVING RECURRENT PERFORMANCE PROBLEMS | 115

FIFTH GUIDELINE FOR DISCIPLINARY ACTION

The final guideline is what is referred to as the *default* characteristic. Disciplinary action should be the last thing done to improve repeated occurrences of problematic performance. It is taken because all the other procedures, such as good training and frequent feedback, have not proven effective. Hence, disciplinary action is a default procedure in that it is relied on when everything else has failed.

SHOW SLIDE 10.8

Slide 10.8: Disciplinary Action as an Indicator of Ineffective Supervision

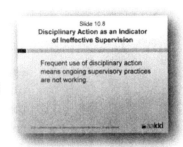

In short, if a supervisor is frequently using disciplinary action month after month, then something is wrong with the overall supervisory approach. In such a case, a reevaluation of the day-to-day supervisory procedures is warranted to determine what the supervisor is not doing correctly.

CONDUCT COMPETENCY CHECK

Conduct the competency check using Competency Check Form 10.1.

Slide 10.1
Summary of Evidence-Based Supervisory Procedures

- Specify performance expectations as staff work behaviors or outcomes.
- Provide performance-based and competency-based training.
- Routinely monitor staff work behavior.
- Provide positive feedback frequently and corrective feedback as needed.

© 2011 American Association on Intellectual and Developmental Disabilities. All rights reserved.

Slide 10.2
Making Work Life Enjoyable and Reducing Discontent

- Interact with staff members in a positive and socially courteous manner.
- Be present in the staff workplace frequently.
- Help out when needed.
- Strive to resolve staff issues of concern.
- Actively work to make disliked tasks more enjoyable for staff members to perform.

© 2011 American Association on Intellectual and Developmental Disabilities. All rights reserved.

Slide 10.3
First Step for Resolving Recurring Performance Problems

Provide corrective feedback.

Slide 10.4
Key Reasons for Recurring Performance Problems and Required Supervisory Action

Lack of skills to perform a work duty	Provide performance-based and competency-based training.
Lack of time or resources	Secure necessary resources or reconsider assignments.
Lack of physical capability to perform a task	Alter a job or consider reassignment.
Lack of motivation to do the task	Provide corrective feedback followed by disciplinary action if needed.

Slide 10.5
Goal of Disciplinary Action

The goal of disciplinary action can be to improve problematic performance *or* to remove the staff member from the agency's employment.

Slide 10.6
Effective Use of Disciplinary Action

1. Routinely practice evidence-based supervision.
2. Be knowledgeable about and adhere to agency policies and procedures for using disciplinary action.
3. Inform superiors prior to taking disciplinary action.
4. Be aware of short- and long-term effects.
5. Rely on disciplinary action only as the default supervisory strategy.

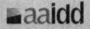

Slide 10.7
Problems With Frequent Reliance on Disciplinary Action

- Staff members adapt and it loses its effectiveness.
- It erodes the overall quality of the work environment.
- It decreases staff motivation to perform job duties in the supervisor's absence.

Slide 10.8
Disciplinary Action as an Indicator of Ineffective Supervision

Frequent use of disciplinary action means ongoing supervisory practices are not working.

MODULE 10 COMPETENCY CHECK
Resolving Recurrent Performance Problems

TRAINER INSTRUCTIONS

- Distribute Competency Check Form 10.1 to each trainee.
- Instruct trainees to respond to both directives on the form.

MASTERY CRITERION

Trainees must correctly respond to both directives.

MODULE 10 COMPETENCY CHECK FORM 10.1

Resolving Recurrent Performance Problems

Trainee name: _____ Date: _____

INSTRUCTIONS

Respond to each of the two following directives:

1. In the box below, draw a line from the *reason* for a performance problem to the most recommended *supervisory action* for resolving the problem.

Reason for a Performance Problem	Supervisory Action
Staff member does not know how to perform a task.	Alter job or consider reassignment.
Lack of time or resources.	Give corrective feedback followed by disciplinary action if needed.
Staff member physically cannot perform task.	Provide training.
Lack of motivation to perform task.	Secure resources or reconsider assignments.

2. Briefly describe five guidelines for using disciplinary action effectively.

   1. _____
   2. _____
   3. _____
   4. _____
   5. _____

FOR TRAINER RECORDING

Did trainee correctly respond to both directives?

   Yes _____   No _____

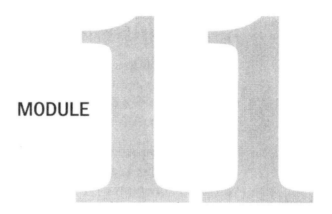

MODULE 11

Putting It All Together
Improving Selected Areas of Staff Performance

The following will be covered on day 2 of training.

Objectives

Upon completion of this module, trainees should be able to do the following:

1. Describe five evidence-based steps for improving an area of staff work performance.
2. Demonstrate with an example how to apply the five steps for improving an area of staff work performance.

Method

1. Presentation and trainee discussion on using evidence-based supervision to improve staff work performance: *5 minutes*
2. Presentation and trainee discussion on systematic steps for improving an area of staff work performance: *10 minutes*
3. Presentation on example of systematic steps for improving an area of staff work performance: *5 minutes*
4. Competency check: *45 minutes*
5. Presentation on summary of evidence-based supervision: *5 minutes*

Competency Check, Materials, and Total Training Time

1. Competency check: Completion of Competency Check Form 11.1
2. Materials
   a. PowerPoint presentation equipment (LCD, computer, curriculum CD) or
   b. Overhead projector and copies of Slides 11.1, 11.2, 11.3, 11.4, and 11.5
   c. Competency Check Form 11.1
3. Total training time: *1 hour and 10 minutes*

Putting It All Together: Improving Selected Areas of Staff Performance

SUPERVISE IN A SYSTEMATIC MANNER

Throughout this training session, a number of procedures have been described that constitute an evidence-based approach to supervision. Each procedure serves a distinct purpose for effectively improving or supporting staff performance, as well as for enhancing staff work enjoyment.

However, the procedures are also intended to be used in conjunction with each other. The supervisory procedures should likewise be practiced in a *systematic* or stepwise fashion.

How the supervisor actions should be practiced systematically is perhaps best illustrated when used to improve an area of staff performance. Every supervisor faces situations in which certain areas of staff performance need significant improvement from time to time.

  QUESTION TRAINEES

Ask trainees to give some examples of areas of staff performance that they would really like to see improved. After several examples have been provided, instruct the trainees to keep those examples in mind during the following discussion and activities.

FOCUS OF THIS SESSION

The focus of this module is on how to use the supervisory procedures we have been discussing in a systematic manner to improve selected areas of staff performance. The intent is to illustrate an evidence-based means of improving the types of performance areas just noted as well as other important areas of work performance that need improvement from time to time.

SHOW SLIDE 11.1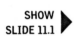

Slide 11.1: Steps for Improving Selected Areas of Staff Work Performance

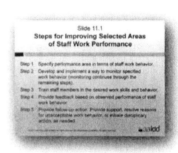

IMPROVING STAFF PERFORMANCE STEP 1

The first step for improving an area of staff performance is to *specify* that area. Remember that "specifying" means the selected area of performance is stated as the staff work behavior that can be observed and counted or measured in a manner such that two people readily agree when the work behavior is occurring.

STEP 2

The second step is to develop and implement a means of *monitoring* the work behavior that constitutes the performance area of concern. This can be done with a checklist or by developing a monitoring tool to count the occurrence of the defined work behaviors. This step in essence provides a baseline evaluation of how well the staff is performing.

STEP 3

The third step is to *train* the staff to perform the identified work behavior or duty with quality. The process of performance-based and competency-based staff training should be implemented as we have emphasized previously. A key point is that training should not be considered complete until each staff member is observed to perform the work duty competently.

Following the staff training session, monitoring should then continue as just described. The results of the monitoring should be used to determine subsequent staff actions. One action that is essentially always needed is to provide *positive feedback* regarding those work behaviors that staff performed correctly during the monitoring. If the monitoring indicates one or more staff did not perform any part of the specified behavior correctly, then *corrective feedback* should be provided.

STEP 4

Providing feedback in this manner represents the fourth step for improving an area of staff performance. Remember, the feedback should be *diagnostic* in nature.

Ask trainees if they remember what constitutes diagnostic feedback. Make sure to point out that "diagnostic" means that the feedback is based on a diagnosis of what was performed correctly and incorrectly. The former staff behavior is followed by positive or supportive feedback and the latter by corrective feedback.

STEP 5

After feedback has been presented, monitoring again continues. Subsequently, Step 5 involves *follow-up* action by the supervisor. If the monitoring indicates a respective staff member is performing the work behaviors appropriately, then the follow-up action entails continuation of positive feedback. Formal recognition or special activities could also be provided if a supervisor wants to provide additional support as discussed in Module 8.

If, however, monitoring indicates at this point that a staff member is not performing satisfactorily, then the follow-up action requires assessment of the reasons for the unsatisfactory performance. Corresponding corrective action should then be taken as discussed in Module 10.

DISCIPLINARY ACTION AS LAST FOLLOW-UP STEP

This step may also involve disciplinary action with the staff but, again, only if all the other supervisory steps have been taken. Most importantly, disciplinary action should be provided only after feedback has been presented at least two or three times for the work behavior of concern.

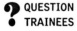

Briefly review the steps on Slide 11.1 by naming them. Then ask trainees if the basic steps are clear or if they have any questions about the steps. Answer any questions posed.

MODULE 11: PUTTING IT ALL TOGETHER

This systematic approach to improving staff performance has a strong evidence base in both research and application to support its effectiveness. It has helped supervisors improve many different areas of staff work performance. It has been used frequently, for example, to increase staff social interactions with clients, improve teaching proficiency, reduce absenteeism, improve paperwork efficiency, and increase choices that the staff provides to clients.

EXAMPLE OF USE OF SUPERVISORY STEPS

Let us show how the approach has been used to improve one of the staff performance areas just noted. Specifically, we will show how the steps have been used to promote the staff's provision of choice opportunities for supported workers with severe disabilities during their work routine.

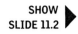

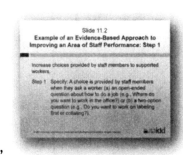

Slide 11.2: Example of Evidence-Based Approach to Improving an Area of Staff Performance—Step 1

The concern in this situation was that the supported workers had minimal or no choice regarding how they completed their work even though agency management had repeatedly stressed the importance of choice opportunities on the clients' quality of life. Using the systematic approach just summarized, the first step the supervisor took was to define the specific staff behavior that represented a choice opportunity for a client. See how choice was defined on this slide as observable staff behavior.

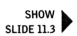

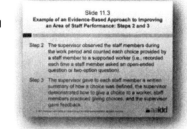

Slide 11.3: Example of Evidence-Based Approach to Improving an Area of Staff Performance—Steps 2 and 3

The second supervisory step involved the supervisor monitoring staff choice behavior during client work periods as illustrated on this slide; the supervisor counted and kept a record of how many choices were provided by each staff member. The third step involved the supervisor meeting with each staff member and training him or her as to what was meant by providing a choice and how to provide choices as also shown on the slide.

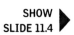

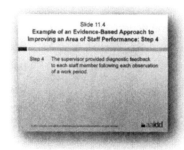

Slide 11.4: Example of Evidence-Based Approach to Improving an Area of Staff Performance—Step 4

After training each staff member, the supervisor then gave diagnostic feedback to the staff after each work period based on the number of choice opportunities each staff provided for the supported workers.

SHOW SLIDE 11.5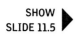

Slide 11.5: Example of Evidence-Based Approach to Improving an Area of Staff Performance—Outcome

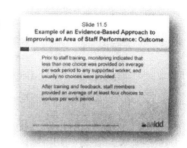

The supervisory process resulted in clear improvement in staff performance. Prior to the supervisor's efforts, staff gave very few if any work choices to the supported workers. Afterward, though, each staff member was giving an average of at least four choices to each supported worker during a work period. Because all the staff members improved their performance once training and feedback were provided, follow-up action (Step 5) simply involved the supervisor continuing to provide periodic feedback to the staff members about their provision of choices to supported workers after subsequent work periods.

REFER TO APPENDIX A

As indicated previously, this same approach to improving staff work performance has been successful with many important work duties.

CONDUCT COMPETENCY CHECK

Conduct the competency check using Competency Check Form 11.1.

QUESTION TRAINEES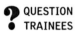

After completing the competency check, ask a representative from one of the trainee groups to summarize each of their steps for improving an area of staff performance. Select a group that you perceived did a good job in completing the competency check based on the previous summaries presented to the class.

SHOW SLIDE 11.1 AGAIN

Slide 11.1: Steps for Improving a Selected Area of Staff Performance

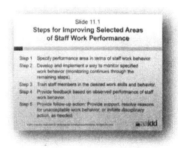

REVIEW SUPERVISORY STEPS

The example provided shows how to use an evidence-based means of supervision to improve staff work performance. To review briefly, the performance area of concern is specified in terms of staff work behavior, that behavior is monitored regularly, staff are trained in the skills to perform the desired work behavior, feedback is provided based on how well staff perform the duty, and follow-up supportive and corrective actions are taken as needed.

EFFECTIVE SUPERVISION IS NOT EASY

Though this approach to improving an area of staff performance is usually quite effective, it is not always easy. It takes time, effort, and persistence on the part of the supervisor.

EFFECTIVE SUPERVISION LEADS TO QUALITY SERVICES

Sometimes the time and effort can be reduced because not all the steps are necessary. Most commonly, a supervisor may know the lack of satisfactory performance is not due to staff not knowing how to perform the duty—the supervisor has seen staff perform adequately when they want to. In this situation, the staff training step can be omitted.

However, usually supervisors still must be willing to work diligently and persist in their efforts. Most supervisors do work hard at their jobs, but often *what* they are doing to impact staff performance is not consistently effective. Using evidence-based means to supervise, as we have discussed throughout this class, tremendously increases the likelihood that a supervisor's efforts will result in quality staff performance. In turn, supports and services provided to agency clients are likely to be of a high quality.

Slide 11.1
Steps for Improving Selected Areas of Staff Work Performance

Step 1 Specify performance area in terms of staff work behavior.

Step 2 Develop and implement a way to monitor specified work behavior (monitoring continues through the remaining steps).

Step 3 Train staff members in the desired work skills and behavior.

Step 4 Provide feedback based on observed performance of staff work behavior.

Step 5 Provide follow-up action: Provide support, resolve reasons for unacceptable work behavior, or initiate disciplinary action, as needed.

Slide 11.2
Example of an Evidence-Based Approach to Improving an Area of Staff Performance: Step 1

Increase choices provided by staff members to supported workers.

Step 1 Specify: A choice is provided by staff members when they ask a worker (a) an open-ended question about how to do a job (e.g., Where do you want to work in the office?) or (b) a two-option question (e.g., Do you want to work on labeling first or collating?).

Slide 11.3
Example of an Evidence-Based Approach to Improving an Area of Staff Performance: Steps 2 and 3

Step 2 The supervisor observed the staff members during the work period and counted each choice provided by a staff member to a supported worker (i.e., recorded each time a staff member asked an open-ended question or two-option question).

Step 3 The supervisor gave to each staff member a written summary of how a choice was defined, the supervisor demonstrated how to give a choice to a worker, staff members practiced giving choices, and the supervisor gave feedback.

© 2011 American Association on Intellectual and Developmental Disabilities. All rights reserved.

Slide 11.4
Example of an Evidence-Based Approach to Improving an Area of Staff Performance: Step 4

Step 4 The supervisor provided diagnostic feedback to each staff member following each observation of a work period.

© 2011 American Association on Intellectual and Developmental Disabilities. All rights reserved.

Slide 11.5
Example of an Evidence-Based Approach to Improving an Area of Staff Performance: Outcome

Prior to staff training, monitoring indicated that less than one choice was provided on average per work period to any supported worker, and usually no choices were provided.

After training and feedback, staff members provided an average of at least four choices to workers per work period.

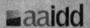

MODULE 11 COMPETENCY CHECK

Putting It All Together: Improving Selected Areas of Staff Performance

TRAINER INSTRUCTIONS

- Distribute Competency Check Form 11.1 to each trainee.
- Instruct the trainees to gather in small groups at their tables.
- Read the instructions at the top of the form.
- Instruct trainees to follow the instructions on the form and jointly determine how to complete each part of Form 11.1.
- Inform trainees that they should stop after completing each part of the form and that they will be asked to share what they completed for that part with the rest of the class before they work on the next part.
- Inform trainees that each person should answer each part of Form 11.1 based on what the group decides and each trainee should turn in his or her completed form at the end.
- Allow no more than 45 minutes for the activity.

SPECIAL TRAINER NOTE

Review each group's answer to each part with the entire class to make sure it is appropriately answered before allowing the group to proceed to the next part. Pay special attention to part 1 to make sure the performance area selected addresses a specific performance area (there may be a tendency for trainees to select areas that are too comprehensive or global; have them focus on a specific area).

MASTERY CRITERION

Each trainee must correctly answer each question on Competency Check Form 11.1 (based on guidelines related to each supervisory procedure discussed in previous modules).

MODULE 11 COMPETENCY CHECK FORM 11.1

Putting It All Together: Improving Selected Areas of Staff Performance

Trainee name: _____ Date: _____

INSTRUCTIONS

Within your group, jointly decide how to answer each of the questions on the following form and complete the form in the following manner. First, jointly decide how to answer question 1, and then each of you record your answer on your form. Stop at that point until you are asked to share your answer with the rest of the class. The entire class will reach a consensus with the trainers regarding whether the question was answered appropriately using guidelines from previous modules (e.g., for Step 4 on staff training, the training procedures must be performance and competency based). Then use the same process for each of the remaining parts (i.e., jointly decide the answer, each of you record the answer on the form, wait at that point until you are asked to share your answer with the rest of the class, and get feedback from the rest of the class and the trainers).

STEPS FOR IMPROVING AN AREA OF STAFF PERFORMANCE

1. Which selected area of staff performance will be improved?

2. How will the area selected in question 1 be defined in terms of staff work behavior that can be observed and counted, and will the group as a whole be able to agree when the work behavior does or does not occur?

3. What system will you use to monitor work behavior? Describe in sufficient detail such that another supervisor could take your description and use it to monitor staff behavior.

4. How will you train staff to perform the work behaviors representing the selected performance area?

5. When and how often will diagnostic feedback be provided to the staff once trained?

6. What other special recognition may be provided for support staff who perform the selected work behaviors in an exemplary manner?

Part III

On-the-Job Competency Checks:
Trainer Instructions and Forms

Trainer Instructions and Forms for On-the-Job Competency Checks

To successfully complete the training requirements of *The Supervisor Training Curriculum*, each supervisory trainee must demonstrate mastery on three competency checks at the trainee's routine work site. The checks involve review of a job duty checklist that the trainee developed, formally observing a staff member's performance of the job duty represented on the checklist, and providing diagnostic feedback to the staff member based on the observed performance. These on-the-job competency checks are intended to be conducted after completion of Modules 1 through 6 of the training and before beginning Module 7. However, the checks can be conducted at any time after completion of the first six modules.

To assist in conducting the on-the-job competency checks, the following information is provided in the remainder of this part: (a) general instructions that should be provided at the end of the last class session prior to conducting the on-the-job competency checks, (b) specific instructions pertaining to each of the three checks (also to be provided in class prior to the competency checks), (c) instructions for trainers concerning how to conduct the competency checks, (d) required trainee mastery criteria for each competency check, and (e) an observation form to be used during the last of the three checks.

General Instructions

The following should be explained to the trainees at the end of the last class session before conducting the on-the-job competency checks. First, a schedule should be developed jointly by the trainee and trainer regarding the date and time to conduct each trainee's competency check at his or her designated work site. The schedule should allow 45 minutes to be spent with each trainee. Second, trainees must be at their respective work sites at the time for the scheduled competency checks. Third, trainees should be very familiar with the job they will be observed to perform and should review the modules (see below) that pertain to each of the three checks. Fourth, three competency checks will be conducted: (a) a review of a job duty checklist that the trainee has developed for use at his or her work site (from Module 3), (b) formal monitoring with the trainer of a staff member's performance of the duty for which the checklist was developed (from Module 4), and (c) trainee provision of diagnostic feedback based on the staff member's performance of the job duty that was monitored (from Module 6).

Next, review the following instructions pertaining to each of the three competency checks.

Specific Instructions for Each Competency Check

Competency Check 1: Review of a Job Duty Checklist

Instruct trainees to review, prior to the on-the-job competency check, Module 3 ("Making Performance Expectations Clear: Job Duty Checklists") in their trainee guide. Explain that each trainee should develop a checklist prior to the scheduled date of the competency check, using the guidelines described in Module 3. Indicate the checklist must pertain to a job duty that one or more staff members is expected to complete regularly. The job duty must also be one that a staff member can perform at the scheduled time of the competency check. Next, explain that the trainer will review the checklist with the trainee to determine if each step is written in a manner that reflects specific work behavior, which can be observed and counted as occurring or not, and that both the trainee and trainer can readily agree if the behavior occurs. Explain further that the trainee should have one copy of the checklist for his or her use and one for the trainer.

Competency Check 2: Formal Monitoring of Staff Performance

Instruct trainees to review, prior to the on-the-job competency check, Module 4 ("Assessing Work Performance: Formal Monitoring") in their trainee guide. Indicate that each trainee will observe a staff member's performance of the job duty for which the job duty checklist was developed as referred to previously, as the trainer simultaneously observes the performance with the same checklist. Instruct trainees that they should practice using the checklist to observe staff performance prior to the competency check to refine and finalize the checklist using the guidelines specified for Competency Check 1. Next, explain that the trainees should arrange for a staff member to perform the designated job duty at the scheduled time for the competency check so that the person's performance can be observed. Inform the trainees that after the observation, the recordings of the trainee on the checklist will be compared to the recordings of the trainer to assess the degree to which the observations and recordings coincided. Also indicate that if satisfactory agreement between the trainee and trainer do not result, then the trainer will work with the trainee to refine the checklist or the monitoring process using the checklist and then repeat the monitoring. Hence, the trainee should be prepared to have the staff member repeat the job duty or have another staff member prepared to perform the duty.

Competency Check 3: Providing Diagnostic Feedback

Instruct trainees to review, prior to the on-the-job competency check, Module 6 ("Improving and Supporting Work Performance: Diagnostic Feedback"). Explain that trainees will be observed providing feedback to the staff member observed in Competency Check 2 following the latter's completion of the job duty. Indicate that the feedback should include each of the seven steps previously practiced in class and represented on Competency Check Form 6.1 from Module 6, and that they should review the steps in their trainee guide (a copy of the feedback form is also included at the end of this part and can be copied and provided to the trainees for their subsequent use). Indicate also that the trainees should practice the seven steps of diagnostic feedback prior to the competency check so that they become very familiar with providing such feedback. Inform them that it is usually helpful to have a copy of the steps with them as they give feedback and that they should have a copy with them during the actual competency check. Finally, explain to the trainees that as with Competency Check 2 on monitoring, if they do not meet the mastery criterion while providing feedback, then they will be asked to provide feedback again following another observation of a staff member's performance (and after the trainer has reviewed the trainee's feedback performance).

Instructions to Trainers for Conducting On-the-Job Competency Checks

When conducting on-the-job competency checks, the trainer should use the following guidelines:

1. Have several copies of the competency check form at the end of this part for providing diagnostic feedback.
2. Arrive at the trainee's work site at the scheduled time.
3. Question the trainee prior to beginning the first competency check to see if he or she has any questions regarding the three checks (reviewing a job duty checklist, monitoring staff performance with the checklist, and providing feedback) and respond to any questions posed.
4. Conduct Competency Checks 1, 2, and 3 in this order and assess trainee performance for each check using the respective mastery criteria presented in the following section.
5. Provide feedback to the trainee following each competency check.
6. Repeat each competency check for which the trainee did not meet the mastery criterion, provide feedback again, and continue the process until the trainee reaches the criterion.

Mastery Criteria for Trainer Use to Evaluate Trainee Performance for Each Competency Check

Competency Check 1: Review of Job Duty Checklist

Review each step on the checklist with the trainee. For each step to be acceptable, it must specify staff behavior to the degree the behavior can be observed and the trainer and the trainee would likely agree if the behavior occurred based on the step specification. Each step of the checklist must be written in this manner.

Competency Check 2: Formal Monitoring of Staff Performance

The trainee's recordings of the staff member's performance on the checklist must agree with the trainer's recordings for at least 80% of the listed steps. An agreement is counted if the trainer and trainee both scored, for a given step, that the staffer performed the behavior constituting the step or both scored that the staffer did not perform the behavior.

Competency Check 3: Providing Diagnostic Feedback

See mastery criterion at the bottom of the following Diagnostic Feedback Monitoring Form.

Observation Form to Use During On-the-Job Competency Check 3: Providing Diagnostic Feedback: Diagnostic Feedback Monitoring Form

1. Begins feedback with positive or empathetic statement:

    Yes _____   No _____

2. Tells staff member at least one work behavior performed correctly:

    Yes _____   No _____

3. Tells staff member at least one work behavior performed incorrectly (if applicable):

    Yes _____   No _____   NA _____

4. Tells staff member specifically how to correct work behavior that was performed incorrectly (if applicable):

    Yes _____   No _____   NA _____

5. Asks staff member if he or she has any questions about the feedback:

    Yes _____   No _____

6. Tells staff member when the performance will be observed again and feedback will be provided:

    Yes _____   No _____

7. Ends feedback with positive or empathetic statement:

    Yes _____   No _____

MASTERY CRITERION FOR TRAINER RECORDING

1. Total number steps scored "Yes": _____
2. Total number steps scored "No": _____
3. Number of "Yes" ÷ (number of "Yes" + number of "No") = _____
   Did trainee receive at least 80% "Yes" recordings on #3 above and complete Step 2 correctly? _____

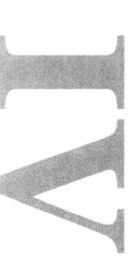

Part IV

Selected Background Readings

Selected Background Readings

The following are readings that describe examples of the background research that provides the evidence base of the supervisory procedures in *The Supervisor Training Curriculum*. The readings are not exhaustive of the total body of research on evidence-based supervision but represent an illustrative sample. The readings are organized according to the main components of supervision as described in the 11 modules of the curriculum. Additionally, several readings are references that pertain to summary overviews of evidence-based approaches to supervising staff performance in the human services.

Specifying Performance Expectations and Monitoring Staff Work Behavior

Dancer, D. D., Braukmann, C. J., Schumaker, J. B., Kirigin, K. A., Willner, A. G., & Wolf, M. M. (1978). The training and validation of behavior observation and description skills. *Behavior Modification, 2*, 113–133.

Epstein, L. H., & Wolff, E. (1978). A multiple baseline analysis of implementing components of the problem-oriented medical record. *Behavior Therapy, 9*, 85–88.

Green, C. W., Canipe, V. C., Way, P. J., & Reid, D. H. (1986). Improving the functional utility and effectiveness of classroom services for students with profound multiple handicaps. *Journal of the Association for Persons With Severe Handicaps, 11*, 162–170.

Greene, B. F., Willis, B. S., Levy, R., & Bailey, J. S. (1978). Measuring client gains from staff-implemented programs. *Journal of Applied Behavior Analysis, 11*, 395–412.

Horner, R. H., Thompsen, L. S., & Storey, K. (1990). Effects of case manager feedback on the quality of individual habilitation plan objectives. *Mental Retardation, 28*, 227–231.

Jones, H. H., Morris, E. K., & Barnard, J. D. (1986). Increasing staff completion of civil commitment forms through instructions and graphed group performance feedback. *Journal of Organizational Behavior Management, 7*(3/4), 29–43.

Lattimore, J., Stephens, T. E., Favell, J. E., & Risley, T. R. (1984). Increasing direct care staff compliance to individualized physical therapy body positioning prescriptions: Prescriptive checklists. *Mental Retardation, 22*, 79–84.

Page, T. J., Christian, J. G., Iwata, B. A., Reid, D. H., Crow, R. E., & Dorsey, M. F. (1981). Evaluating and training interdisciplinary teams in writing IPP goals and objectives. *Mental Retardation, 19*, 25–27.

Parsons, M. B., Cash, V. B., & Reid, D. H. (1989). Improving residential treatment services: Implementation and norm-referenced evaluation of a comprehensive management system. *Journal of Applied Behavior Analysis, 22*, 143–156.

Thompson, T. J., Thornhill, C. A., Realon, R. E., & Ervin, K. M. (1991). Improving accuracy in documentation of restrictive interventions by direct-care personnel. *Mental Retardation, 29*, 201–205.

Van den Pol, R. A., Reid, D. H., & Fuqua, R. W. (1983). Peer training of safety-related skills to institutional staff: Benefits for trainers and trainees. *Journal of Applied Behavior Analysis, 16*, 139–156.

Staff Training

Adams, G. L., Tallon, R. J., & Rimmell, P. (1980). A comparison of lecture versus role-playing in the training of the use of positive reinforcement. *Journal of Organizational Behavior Management, 2*(3), 205–212.

Burch, M. R., Reiss, M. M., & Bailey, J. S. (1987). A competency-based "hands-on" training package for direct care staff. *Journal of the Association for Persons With Severe Handicaps, 12*, 67–71.

Demchak, M. A. (1987). A review of behavioral staff training in special education settings. *Education and Training in Mental Retardation, 22*, 205–217.

Engelman, K. K., Altus, D. E., Mosier, M. C., & Mathews, R. M. (2003). Brief training to promote the use of less intrusive prompts by nursing assistants in a dementia care unit. *Journal of Applied Behavior Analysis, 36,* 129–132.

Lavie, T., & Sturmey, P. (2002). Training staff to conduct a paired-stimulus preference assessment. *Journal of Applied Behavior Analysis, 35,* 209–211.

Macurik, K. M., O'Kane, N. P., Malanga, P., & Reid, D. H. (2008). Video training of support staff in intervention plans for challenging behavior: Comparison with live training. *Behavioral Interventions, 23,* 143–163.

Miles, N. I., & Wilder, D. A. (2009). The effects of behavioral skills training on caregiver implementation of guided compliance. *Journal of Applied Behavior Analysis, 42,* 405–410.

Parsons, M. B., & Reid, D. H. (1999). Training basic teaching skills to paraeducators of students with severe disabilities: A one-day program. *Teaching Exceptional Children, 31,* 48–54.

Parsons, M. B., Reid, D. H., & Green, C. W. (1996). Training basic teaching skills to community and institutional support staff for people with severe disabilities: A one-day program. *Research in Developmental Disabilities, 17,* 467–485.

Reid, D. H., Rotholz, D. A., Parsons, M. B., Morris, L., Braswell, B., Green, C. W., & Schell, R. M. (2003). Training human service supervisors in aspects of positive behavior support: Evaluation of a statewide, performance-based program. *Journal of Positive Behavioral Interventions, 2,* 170–178.

Sarokoff, R. A., & Sturmey, P. (2004). The effects of behavioral skills training on staff implementation of discrete-trial teaching. *Journal of Applied Behavior Analysis, 37,* 535–538.

Schepis, M. M., Reid, D. H., Ownbey, J., & Clary, J. (2003). Training preschool staff to promote cooperative participation among young children with severe disabilities and their classmates. *Research and Practice in Severe Disabilities, 28,* 37–42.

Schepis, M. M., Reid, D. H., Ownbey, J., & Parsons, M. B. (2001). Training support staff to embed teaching within natural routines of young children with disabilities in an inclusive preschool. *Journal of Applied Behavior Analysis, 34,* 313–328.

Improving and Supporting Work Performance: Feedback

Alavosius, M. P., & Sulzer-Azaroff, B. (1990). Acquisition and maintenance of health-care routines as a function of feedback density. *Journal of Applied Behavior Analysis, 23,* 151–162.

Alvero, A. M., Bucklin, B. R., & Austin, J. (2001). An objective review of the effectiveness and essential characteristics of performance feedback in organizational settings. *Journal of Organizational Behavior Management, 21,* 3–29.

Brown, K. M., Willis, B. S., & Reid, D. H. (1981). Differential effects of supervisor verbal feedback and feedback plus approval on institutional staff performance. *Journal of Organizational Behavior Management, 3*(1), 57–68.

Codding, R. S., Feinberg, A. B., Dunn, E. K., & Pace, G. M. (2005). Effects of immediate performance feedback on implementation of behavior support plans. *Journal of Applied Behavior Analysis, 38,* 205–219.

Codding, R. S., Livanis, A., Pace, G. M., & Vaca, L. (2008). Using performance feedback to improve treatment integrity of classwide behavior plans: An investigation of observer reactivity. *Journal of Applied Behavior Analysis, 41,* 417–422.

DiGennaro, F. D., Martens, B. K., & Kleinmann, A. E. (2007). A comparison of performance feedback procedures on teachers' treatment implementation integrity and students' inappropriate behavior in special education classrooms. *Journal of Applied Behavior Analysis, 40,* 447–461.

Green, C. W., Rollyson, J. H., Passante, S. C., & Reid, D. H. (2002). Maintaining proficient supervisor performance with direct support personnel: An analysis of two management approaches. *Journal of Applied Behavior Analysis, 35,* 205–208.

Parsons, M. B., & Reid, D. H. (1995). Training residential supervisors to provide feedback for maintaining staff teaching skills with people who have severe disabilities. *Journal of Applied Behavior Analysis, 28,* 317–322.

Wilson, P. G., Reid, D. H., & Korabek-Pinkowski, C. A. (1991). Analysis of public verbal feedback as a staff management procedure. *Behavioral Residential Treatment, 6,* 263–277.

Promoting Work Enjoyment and Reducing Discontent

Green, C. W., Reid, D. H., Passante, S., & Canipe, V. (2008). Changing less-preferred duties to more-preferred: A potential strategy for improving supervisor work enjoyment. *Journal of Organizational Behavior Management, 28,* 90–109.

Parsons, M. B. (1998). A review of procedural acceptability in organizational behavior management. *Journal of Organizational Behavior Management, 18,* 173–190.

Parsons, M. B., Reid, D. H., & Crow, R. E. (2003). The best and worst ways to motivate staff in community agencies: A brief survey of supervisors. *Mental Retardation, 41,* 96–102.

Reid, D. H., & Parsons, M. B. (1995). Comparing choice versus questionnaire measures of acceptability of a staff training procedure. *Journal of Applied Behavior Analysis, 28,* 95–96.

Reid, D. H., & Parsons, M. B. (1996). A comparison of staff acceptability of immediate versus delayed feedback in staff training. *Journal of Organizational Behavior Management, 16,* 35–47.

Summaries of Evidence-Based Approaches to Supervision

Harchik, A. E., Sherman, J. A., Sheldon, J. B., & Strouse, M. C. (1992). Ongoing consultation as a method of improving performance of staff members in a group home. *Journal of Applied Behavior Analysis, 25,* 599–610.

Kneringer, M. J., & Page, T. J. (1999). Improving staff nutritional practices in community-based group homes: Evaluation, training, and management. *Journal of Applied Behavior Analysis, 32,* 221–224.

Parsons, M. B., Rollyson, J. H., & Reid, D. H. (2004). Improving day treatment services for adults with severe disabilities: A norm-referenced application of outcome management. *Journal of Applied Behavior Analysis, 37,* 365–377.

Reid, D. H. (Ed.). (1998). *Organizational behavior management and developmental disabilities services: Accomplishments and future directions.* Binghamton, NY: Haworth Press.

Reid, D. H., Green, C. W., & Parsons, M. B. (2003). An outcome management program for extending advances in choice research into choice opportunities for supported workers with severe multiple disabilities. *Journal of Applied Behavior Analysis, 36,* 575–578.

Reid, D. H., & Parsons, M. B. (2002). *Working with staff to overcome challenging behavior among people who have severe disabilities: A guide for getting support plans carried out.* Morganton, NC: Habilitative Management Consultants.

Reid, D. H., & Parsons, M. B. (2006). *Motivating human service staff: Supervisory strategies for maximizing work effort and enjoyment* (2nd ed.). Morganton, NC: Habilitative Management Consultants.

Reid, D. H., Parsons, M. B., Lattimore, L. P., Towery, D. L., & Reade, K. K. (2005). Improving staff performance through clinician application of outcome management. *Research in Developmental Disabilities, 26,* 101–116.

Williams, W. L., Vittorio, T. D., & Hausherr, L. (2002). A description and extension of a human services management model. *Journal of Organizational Behavior Management, 22,* 47–71.

If you would like to receive the Power Point slides that accompany this curriculum, please email your request to books@aaidd.org.

CPSIA information can be obtained at www.ICGtesting.com
Printed in the USA
BVOW021808081011

273081BV00004B/1/P

9 781935 304081